Refresh
Revive
Restore
10-Day Detox

Refresh
Revive
Restore
10-Day Detox

Dr. Cobi Slater,
PhD, DNM, RHT, NNCP, RNCP

PhD Natural Health Sciences

Board Certified Doctor of Natural Medicine

Registered Herbal Therapist

Natural Nutritional Consulting Practitioner

Registered Nutritional Consulting Practitioner

XULON PRESS

Xulon Press
2301 Lucien Way #415
Maitland, FL 32751
407.339.4217
www.xulonpress.com

Printed in the United States of America.

Dr. Cobi Slater can be reached at www.drcobi.com

ISBN-13: 9781545625262

Table of Contents

It's time to get started!
Refresh Revive Restore
10-Day Detox

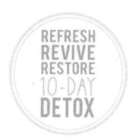

Welcome to the Refresh Revive Restore 10-Day Detox

Thank you so much for making the decision to do the 10 Day Detox. I cannot tell you how excited I am to guide you on your health journey to improved energy, better digestion, clearer skin, weight loss and so much more!

As a Dr. of Natural Medicine, Clinical Nutritionist, Medical Herbalist and PhD in Natural Health Sciences who works with thousands of patients, I am on a mission to help people heal naturally.

In as little as 3, days you should start to experience the positive benefits of the **Refresh Revive Restore 10-Day Detox:**

- ✓ Increased energy and motivation
- ✓ Decreased cravings

- ✓ Improved mood
- ✓ Healthier digestion
- ✓ Rejuvenated sleep
- ✓ Diminished brain fog
- ✓ Clearer skin

I do not want you to feel overwhelmed by this detox. It is not meant to be difficult or expensive. Detoxing is about eating real, healthy and whole foods. It can really be that simple!

Some of you might find it too challenging to implement the full detox. If this is the case for you, then start with smaller steps. Just choosing to add one meal to your diet can make the biggest impact or you can work on one category at a time. For example, begin by improving your snacks and then move onto a healthier breakfast and so on. Go slowly and implement a few things and you will start to feel better in no time.

There are many delicious recipes in my detox guide that are suitable for both vegans and meat eaters. If you are looking for additional recipe inspiration, then head on over to my website at drcobi.com and you will find many more! Plus, there are many great articles on weight loss, detoxification, digestion, natural beauty and hormones for your information.

I am so happy to be along this journey with you, so let's officially get started!

The 10-Day Detox Guidebook includes the following information:

- 10-Day Refresh Revive Restore Detox Guide
- 10-Day Refresh Revive Restore Detox MenuPlan and Recipes
- Cleansing and Detox Questionnaire

- 10 Day Supplement Guide
- 10 Day Weight Tracker
- Kitchen Clean Out Cheat Sheet
- Superfood Cheat Sheet
- Detox Your Home
- Detox Your Hormones
- Detox Your Mind

The Refresh Revive Restore 10-Day Detox is a great start to get you on your way to optimal health. Everything you need to be successful is included in the Refresh Revive Restore Detox Guide.

Please join the Dr Cobi's Insider's Group on Facebook to post your questions, receive great tips and to share your accomplishments.   You will also get dibs on some of my exclusive online health programs as they launch. Stay tuned as I unveil new and exciting programs every season that will help you to feel fantastic! Make sure to sign up for my complimentary monthly newsletter at drcobi.com which includes helpful wellness information to enable you to continue your journey to optimal health.

Be Well,
Dr Cobi.

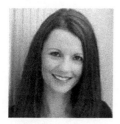

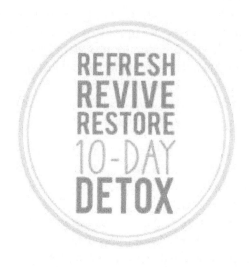

Refresh Revive Restore
10-Day Detox

www.drcobi.com

Medical Disclaimer

All information contained within this Refresh Revive Restore 10-Day Detox is for informational purposes only. It is not intended to diagnose, treat, cure or prevent health problems. It is not intended to replace the advice of a qualified medical practitioner, health practitioner or fitness professional. No action should be taken solely on the contents of this recipe book. Always consult your physician or qualified health professional on any matters regarding your health as well as any opinions expressed in this program.

The information provided within this Refresh Revive Restore 10-Day Detox is believed to be accurate based on the best judgment of the author but the reader is responsible for consulting with his or her own health professional on any health matters. We do not assume liability for the information contained within this detox book, be it direct, indirect, consequential, special, exemplary or any other subsequent damages. It is advisable to consult your physician before changing your diet, starting an exercise program or taking supplements of any kind.

Refresh Revive Restore 10-Day Detox Guide

Here is how the **Refresh Revive Restore 10-Day Detox** works:

1. Fill in the **Detox Questionnaire** to determine your toxic status.

2. Use the **Kitchen Clean Out** cheat sheet to remove processed and tempting foods. Fill a garbage bag with the food and deliver it to the nearest food bank.

3. Follow the **3-Day Liquid Cleanse Meal Plan** for the first 3 days of the Refresh Revive Restore 10-Day Detox.

4. Choose the **Vegan/Vegetarian or the Protein 7-Day Detox Meal Plan** to follow for the remaining 7 days of the Refresh Revive Restore 10-Day Detox.

5. Enjoy snacks from the **Refresh Revive Restore 10-Day Detox Snack List**. If you feel hungry throughout the 10-day detox, including the first 3-Day Liquid Cleanse, choose a snack to have in between meals.

6. Use the **Detox Your Home Guide** to eliminate harmful toxins in your living environment.

7. Use the **Detox Your Hormones Guide** to switch to natural beauty and skin care products that won't cause hormone imbalances.

8. Use the **Detox Your Mind Guide** to free yourself from negative thinking patterns that cause internal toxic buildup.

9. **Partner up!** Research shows that making nutritional changes are more successful when done with others for accountability.

10. **Move your body.** Make a commitment to move your body for at least 30 minutes per day. Activities may include walking, jogging, group fitness classes, spinning, stretching etc.

11. Join and share your experiences in **Dr Cobi's Insider Facebook Group**!

What is Detoxification?

Detoxification is the process of resting, cleansing and nourishing the body from the inside. By removing and eliminating toxins and then feeding your body with healthy nutrients, detoxifying can help protect you from diseases and renew your ability to maintain optimum health.

Give your liver some love!

- Your liver is your #1 detoxifying organ. It has over 500 functions!

- It produces bile (which helps us excrete toxins), regulates carbohydrate metabolism, assists in hormone breakdown and detoxifies **EVERYTHING** we get exposed to in our daily lives.

Action Steps for Optimal Liver Health

1. Start the day with ½ lemon squeezed into 1 cup of warm water.

2. Consume half your body weight in ounces of filtered water daily.

3. Increase fiber consumption to 35 grams per day to assist in the elimination of fat soluble toxins. Choose high fiber foods such as ground flax seeds,

psyllium, apple pectin, rice bran, beet fiber, oat fiber and chia seeds.

4. Consume liver cleansing foods such as beets, bitter greens, apples, lemons, garlic, onions, cabbage, broccoli, Brussels sprouts, kale, collards and cauliflower.

5. Use liver cleansing herbs such as Dandelion root, Artichoke, Milk thistle, Burdock root and Turmeric *(See the 10-Day Detox Supplement Guide for the best Liver Detoxifying Supplements).*

6. Detox the liver with Alpha lipoic acid, Calcium D-Glucarate, NAC, Selenium, Choline and Methionine *(See the 10-Day Detox Supplement Guide for the best Liver Detoxifying Supplements).*

7. Drink liver detoxifying tea with dandelion root, nettle root, red clover, licorice root, burdock root and cleavers.

8. Support the digestion with probiotics and digestive enzymes. *(See the 10-Day Detox Supplement Guide for the best Digestive Support Supplements).*

9. Avoid toxic foods such as sugar, processed foods, refined carbohydrates, pesticides, hydrogenated fats and artificial sugars.

10. Avoid smoking, alcohol, caffeine, pop and energy drinks.

CLEANSING AND DETOX QUESTIONNAIRE

ARE YOU TOXIC?

Have you ever wondered what it would be like to wake up feeling invigorated with a passion and joy to face the day? Imagine going through the day without the aches and pains, fatigue, headaches, depression and all of those symptoms that are preventing you from optimal health. Can you envision yourself full of abundant energy and free from the symptoms that drag you down? If you can't, you could be experiencing an accumulation of toxins in your body. Each year the average person in North America is exposed to 14 pounds of food preservatives, pesticide and herbicide residues. The toxic load on our bodies is increasing every year. If not eliminated, the toxic substances stored in our bodies have detrimental health effects and can lead to chronic disease and cancer. Detoxification is one of the central concepts of natural healing. Cleansing on a regular basis aids in the elimination and neutralization of toxic wastes and helps to revitalize the natural functions of the body.

ARE YOU EXPERIENCING ANY OF THE FOLLOWING?

- ✓ Headaches
- ✓ Eczema/Psoriasis
- ✓ Stomach cramps
- ✓ Constipation
- ✓ Allergies
- ✓ Joint pain

- ✓ Diarrhea
- ✓ Frequent colds
- ✓ Fatigue
- ✓ Acne
- ✓ Slow healing
- ✓ Muscle aches
- ✓ Gas/Bloating
- ✓ Weight gain
- ✓ Fogginess
- ✓ Depression
- ✓ Heartburn/Indigestion
- ✓ Food cravings

If you are experiencing any of these symptoms, going on a detoxification program will have a tremendous impact on your health. Many people shy away from cleansing and detoxing because they think they will have to starve themselves. The opposite is actually true. During a detox, you can eat as much of the recommended foods as you like. You can eliminate an abundance of toxins from your body by simply removing the top allergenic and inflammatory foods from your diet for a minimum of 10 days. In addition, incorporating the necessary herbs, vitamins, amino acids and nutrients are essential steps for cleansing.

Some of the changes that my patients have experienced as a result of cleansing are remarkable. These changes have included weight loss, increased energy, uplifted moods, enhanced immunity, complete healing from digestive symptoms, reduction of arthritic symptoms and clearing of skin problems to name a few.

DETOXIFICATION QUESTIONNAIRE[1]

Signs and symptoms of liver toxicity are diverse. In order to determine if your liver is showing signs of stress, the following questionnaire will help to clarify your need for detoxification. Answer the questions before and after the 10-Day Detox to determine how well your body has responded to the detox.

Point Scale

0- Never or almost never have the symptom

1- Occasionally have it, effect is not severe

2- Occasionally have it, effect is severe

3- Frequently have it, effect is not severe

4- Frequently have it, effect is severe

Head	Skin	Weight
Headaches	Acne	Binge or compulsive eating/drinking
Dizziness	Hives, rashes, dry skin	Craving certain foods
Insomnia	Hair loss	Excessive weight/ Underweight
Faintness	Flushing, hot flashes, excessive sweating	Water retention
Total	Total	Total
Eyes	**Heart**	**Energy/Activity**
Watery or Itchy eyes	Chest pain	Fatigue, sluggishness

[1] FLT Tools/Metagenics/Detox Questionnaire

Swollen, reddened or sticky eyelids	Irregular or skipped heart beat	Apathy, lethargy
Bags or dark circles under eyes	Rapid heart beat	Hyperactivity
Blurred or tunnel vision	Pounding heart beat	Restlessness
Total	Total	Total
Ears	**Lungs**	**Emotions**
Itchy ears	Chest congestion	Mood swings
Ear aches, ear infections	Asthma, bronchitis	Anxiety, fear, nervousness
Drainage from ear	Shortness of breath	Anger, irritability, aggressiveness
Ringing in ears, hearing loss	Difficulty breathing	Depression
Total	Total	Total
Nose	**Digestive Tract**	**Mind**
Stuffy nose	Nausea, vomiting	Poor memory
Sinus problems	Diarrhea, constipation	Confusion, poor comprehension
Hay fever	Bloating, gas, belching	Difficulty making decisions
Sneezing attacks	Heartburn	Stuttering, slurred speech

Excessive mucous formation	Intestinal/Stomach pain	Poor physical coordination
		Learning disability
		Poor concentration
Total	Total	Total
Mouth/ Throat	**Joints/Muscle**	**Other**
Chronic coughing	Pain, aches in joints	Frequent illness
Gagging, throat clearing	Arthritis	Frequent or urgent urination
Sore throat, hoarseness, loss of voice	Stiffness or limitation of movement	Genital itch or discharge
Swollen or discolored tongue, gums, lips	Feeling of weakness or tiredness	
Canker sores	Pain or aches in muscles	
Total	Total	Total

INTERPRETATION:

Above 50 - **High**

15-49 - **Moderate**

Below 14 - **Low**

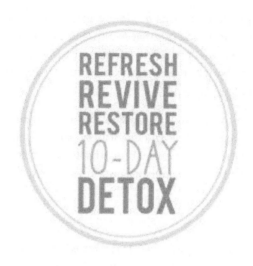

10-Day Supplement Guide

The supplements in this guide are intended to give you a basic foundation for optimal health and detoxification. In order the keep the detoxification pathways working efficiently, the body's main systems need to be supported with the correct nutrients.

This list provides general guidelines for supplements that would be beneficial for the majority of people. Taking these supplements will help to encourage health and detoxification but they are not a compulsory part of the detox.

Many of the recommended products can be purchased from the online store at http://store.drcobi.com/

Use the discount code "10 Day Detox" to receive a 10% discount on all of the recommended products!

The following supplements are suggestions. If you are taking any prescription medications, you should discuss adding in supplements with your pharmacist and/or medical doctor first.

Greens Powder

This is a great option that can be used almost like a multivitamin. A good quality greens product will contain a high number of minerals (a common deficiency in most people), plus a large amount of vitamins and antioxidants. In addition, Greens are very alkalizing which is crucial for strengthening the immune system and keeping your body in the perfect acid-alkaline balance.

Taking a greens product does not take the place of actually eating green veggies. You would take the greens as well as eating all of your delicious green vegetables.

Product recommendations

Paleo Greens- Designs for Health (1 scoop per day)

Greens Powder- Botanica (1 scoop per day)

Probiotics

These are the "good" bacteria that live within your digestive tract. They help to ensure that the "bad" bacteria stay at optimal levels. They also support digestion, keep the immune system healthy (70% of your immune system is actually located in your gut) and enable healthy hormone production.

The use of antibiotics destroys much of your "good" bacteria. Other lifestyle factors such as stress and poor diet lead to less than optimal levels of "good" bacteria. You would benefit from supplementing with probiotics if you are experiencing digestive symptoms such as gas, bloating, constipation or diarrhea, have a lowered immune system or lack overall vitality.

Product recommendations

Ultra Flora Balance - Metagenics (1 capsule on an empty stomach)-general support

Ultra Flora Intensive - Metagenics (1 capsule on an empty stomach)-specific for gas and bloating

HMF IBS - Seroyal (1 capsule on an empty stomach) - specific for symptoms of Irritable Bowel Syndrome

Digestive Enzymes

Digestive enzymes assist in the breakdown of carbohydrates, proteins and fats from food. It is then turned into energy and raw materials to be used in all processes in the body.

The body has the ability to make the enzymes the body needs. In addition, most healthy foods in their raw form have naturally occurring enzymes within them to assist in the process. Factors that affect the body's ability to carry out enzyme production include over consuming processed foods, stress, certain medications as well as the aging process.

Taking digestive enzymes as a supplement can assist the body in breaking down food while you are improving your diet and lifestyle to eventually bring the body's own production of enzymes back into balance.

Product recommendations

GI Digest (vegan)-Douglas Labs (take 1 capsule with each meal)

Ultrazyme-Douglas Labs (take 1 capsule with each meal)

BioLivX

BioLivX contains a variety of nutrients and herbs with proven benefits for protecting and enhancing liver function as well as supporting all detoxification pathways.

Benefits of BioLivX:

- ✓ Specific blend of nutrients and traditional herbs designed to promote healthy liver tissue
- ✓ Contains sodium glucuronate, a key nutritional substance used by the liver to bind toxins
- ✓ Intense liver support

✓ Promotes healthy detoxification of liver toxins and hormone excess

✓ Antioxidant protection neutralizing free radical damage

✓ Reduces oxidative stress and its effects on the body

Take 1 capsule 3 times daily with food until finished. Do not combine with blood pressure medications, blood thinners, during pregnancy or breastfeeding.

Pure Lean Vegan Protein Powder

Pure Lean by Pure Encapsulations is a natural, powdered supplement that provides vegetarian protein, fiber and Omega 3's and is intended to promote weight management.

Eating a protein-rich diet may aid in weight management as protein has been shown to satisfy hunger longer than carbohydrates or fats. In addition, protein may also help to promote a leaner body composition. Pure Lean also contains fiber which reduces cravings as well as appetite. Pure Lean contains Omega 3's which may help to increase your body's metabolism because Omega 3's have the potential ability to support your natural inflammation response. This vegan protein powder also includes other ingredients for the promotion of overall health because it contains minerals and antioxidant-rich fruits.

Add 1 scoop one to two times per day into a smoothie as a meal replacement or snack.

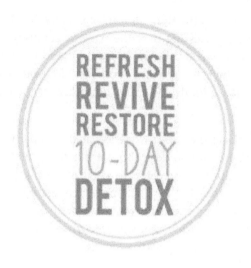

Weight Loss Tracker

Please know that the **Refresh Revive Restore 10-Day Detox** is not about obsessing over the scale or counting calories. Instead, this is about being mindful around food and discovering which foods really work best for you. The most nutrient dense foods will bring nourishment to your body and mind as a whole.

The one thing that does work for many people is to have accountability. If you desire to use this document for your accountability, please feel free to weigh and measure yourself on day 1 of the 10-Day Detox and then again on the final day. I have found that the scale is not always an accurate portrayal of the results that you are achieving. Many people will lose weight very quickly; whereas others will lose inches before the scale even moves.

Feel free to use this chart throughout your entire transformation program or feel free to never step on the scale or pick up a tape measure at all during this detox. The choice is yours. This detox is for you to achieve a feeling of peace with food while losing weight by eating delicious foods and not feeling deprived.

Important note: We are all different in the way that we lose weight. Do not stress about the scale or numbers. Stress is a major reason why we do not lose weight. The more stress there is, the more cortisol (the stress hormone) is secreted which can then lead to additional weight gain!

It is most accurate to weigh and measure first thing in the morning.

Body Part	Day 1	Day 4	Day 7	Day 10
Upper Arm				
Bust				
Waist				
Upper Abdomen				
Lower Abdomen/ Hips				
Upper thigh				
Above the knee				
Total				
	Inches Released			
	Total Inches Released			
Enter Weight on this line				
	Pounds Released			
	Total Pounds Released			

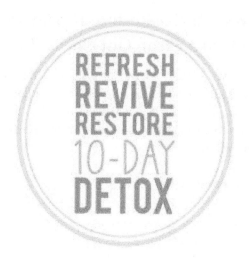

Kitchen Clean Out
Cheat Sheet

Refresh Revive Restore 10-Day Detox Kitchen Clean Out Cheat Sheet

In order to set yourself up for success, you will need to surround yourself with healthy choices. This guide will help you to toss out certain foods that are not health promoting and give you suggestions on how to replace them with healthier options.

Vegetables and Fruit

Toss Out: over processed, low nutrient content fruits and vegetables (canned mixed vegetables, canned fruit, fruit juices and fruit cocktails).

Choose: fresh local or organic produce whenever possible. If buying all organic is not in your budget, look at the Environmental Working Group (EWG) Shoppers Guide to Pesticides to learn about the Dirty Dozen https://www.ewg.org/foodnews/.**This will help you to** invest in the most important organic choices according to the amount of pesticides. The fruits and vegetables on **"The Dirty Dozen"** list, when conventionally grown, tested positive for at least 47 different chemicals with some testing positive for as many as 67. For produce on the "dirty" list, you should definitely **go organic**. "The Dirty Dozen" list includes:

1. Celery
2. Peaches
3. Strawberries
4. Apples
5. Domestic blueberries

6. Nectarines

7. Sweet bell peppers

8. Spinach, kale and collard greens

9. Cherries

10. Potatoes

11. Imported grapes

12. Lettuce

All the produce on "**The Clean 15**" bore little to no traces of pesticides and is safe to consume in non-organic form. This list includes:

1. Onions

2. Avocados

3. Sweet corn

4. Pineapples

5. Mango

6. Sweet peas

7. Asparagus

8. Kiwi fruit

9. Cabbage

10. Eggplant

11. Cantaloupe

12. Watermelon

13. Grapefruit

14. Sweet potatoes

15. Sweet onions

✓ Fresh vegetables: onion, garlic, yam, potato, carrot, beet, radish, squash, rutabaga, leafy greens, kale, arugula, Swiss chard, spinach, watercress, tomato, cabbage, lettuce, celery, broccoli and others in season. Eat a rainbow!

✓ Sprouts and microgreens: sunflower sprouts, buckwheat sprouts, alfalfa sprouts, pea shoots etc.

✓ Frozen vegetables: kale, spinach, rapini, peas and corn

✓ Tomato sauce and paste (look for cans that are BPA free or in glass jars and also do not have sugar in the ingredients)

✓ Fresh fruit in season as well as limited amounts of nutrition packed tropical fruit like papaya, pineapple, mango and bananas

✓ Frozen berries and other mixed fruits

✓ Lemons and limes

✓ Dried fruit (figs, dates, apricots, apples, currants, raisins, goji berries, coconut, etc. - buy unsulphured and organic if possible)

Whole Grain Products

Toss Out: white flour and whole wheat flour products

Choose: a variety of the whole grain gluten-free products below.

1. Gluten free flours: brown rice, teff, quinoa, coconut, almond meal and buckwheat

2. Brown rice: long-grain, short-grain, basmati, jasmine and wild rice

3. Grains in whole form: quinoa, millet, steel cut oats, buckwheat, teff and amaranth

4. Hot cereals for porridge: oats, quinoa, brown rice and teff

Beans and Bean Products

Toss Out: low quality canned beans that contain table salt, preservatives and BPA in the lining of the can.

Choose: dried peas and beans and cook from scratch whenever possible but for convenience use organic frozen or BPA- free canned beans and peas.

1. Try some of these: green and yellow split peas, kidney beans, black beans, chick peas, red and green lentils, navy beans, mung beans, adzuki beans as well as white beans.

2. When choosing canned beans Eden Organics beans are an excellent choice as they contain sea salt rather than table salt and have no BPA in the tin's lining. Go to www.edenorganics.com for over 900 recipe ideas!

3. When using soy products always choose organic (almost all non-organic soy is genetically modified). Organic and fermented or sprouted soy products are even better (sprouted - tofu, fermented - tempeh and miso).

Meat, Meat Products and Fish

Toss Out: factory farmed meats, meats raised with antibiotics and hormones, grain fed meats, lunch meats preserved with nitrates, meat products with additional processed ingredients, farmed fish and seafood.

Choose: naturally raised and/or organic meats (grass-fed, antibiotic/hormone free), meat products that are 100% meat with no added ingredients (spices are okay), lunch meats preserved without nitrates, wild caught fish and seafood.

Nuts, Seeds, Fats & Oils

Toss Out: conventional nut butters made with hydrogenated oils and sugar, roasted nuts and seeds (some are okay- just make sure they are dry roasted or roasted in a high quality oil such as coconut oil), highly refined oils such as canola, sunflower, safflower, cottonseed, peanut and butter made from factory farmed dairy.

Choose: nut and seed butters made without added sugar or hydrogenated fats (they should only have one ingredient on the label e.g.- almond butter should only contain almonds), raw nuts and seeds as well as high quality oils listed below.

1. Nuts (raw almonds, cashews, walnuts, pecans, pine nuts, organic peanuts, brazil nuts etc.)
2. Nut butters (almond, hazelnut, cashew etc.)
3. Seeds (sunflower, pumpkin, hemp, sesame, hemp, flax and chia- look for sprouted versions)
4. Tahini (sesame paste)
5. Extra virgin olive oil (good for low heat cooking)
6. Coconut oil (good for higher heat cooking/baking)
7. Hemp seed oil (do not cook with this)
8. Flax oil (do not cook with this)
9. Organic grass-fed butter and ghee (good for cooking/baking)
10. Other cold-pressed oils - walnut, sesame, avocado and grape seed

Dairy and Substitutes

Toss Out: Traditional dairy products produced from factory-farmed dairy, dairy substitutes that are sweetened or contain an abundance of processed ingredients and preservatives as well as factory-farmed eggs.

Choose: Organic, grass-fed dairy products, dairy substitutes that are unsweetened and have minimal ingredients.

Note: Dairy may not be appropriate for everyone.

1. Milk (organic grass-fed cow, goat, sheep)
2. Cheese (organic dairy, raw if possible)
3. Yogurt and kefir (organic and unsweetened)
4. Butter and Ghee (organic, grass-fed)
5. Alternative milks (dairy substitutes): almond, hemp, coconut, cashew and brown rice
6. Organic or farm fresh eggs

Herbs, Spices, Seasonings, Condiments and Miscellaneous

Toss Out: Highly processed condiments and seasonings that contain white sugar, preservatives, table salt and low quality oils, spices as well as seasonings that contain MSG.

Choose: Minimally processed condiments and seasonings with better quality ingredients. Use fresh and dried herbs and spices, vinegars and oils for flavor more often in replacement of sauces.

Herbs and Spices:

1. Fresh herbs - parsley, basil, thyme, oregano, tarragon, coriander, sage, etc.

2. Dried herbs and spices (make sure you buy non-irradiated - Frontier is a good brand): Allspice, Basil, Cayenne, Celery seed, Chili powder, Cinnamon, Cloves, ground Coriander, Cumin, Curry, Dill, Ginger, Nutmeg, Mustard powder, Oregano, Paprika, Parsley, Rosemary, Sage, Tarragon, Thyme, Turmeric etc.

Seasonings and Condiments

1. Tamari or Braggs Liquid Seasoning
2. Coconut Sauce (Soy-free sauce)
3. Mustard made with apple cider vinegar and sea salt
4. Bottled salad dressings made with high quality oils and natural sweeteners (making your own is the best choice)
5. Sauerkraut (raw/unpasteurized)
6. Natural mayonnaise (made with high quality oils and without white sugar)
7. Vinegars: balsamic, apple cider, rice and red wine
8. Red pepper flakes and chipotle peppers
9. Celtic sea salt, Himalayan salt and Herbamare
10. Dulse flakes, kelp or dulse shakers
11. Nutritional yeast (gives a cheesy flavour without the dairy)

Miscellaneous

1. Arrowroot powder (to use instead of corn starch as a thickening agent)

2. Real vanilla extract (Frontier Organic is a good brand)

3. Aluminum- free baking soda/powder

Sweeteners

Toss: white sugar and anything that contains it as well as anything that contains high fructose corn syrup, artificial sweeteners (aspartame, Splenda, NutraSweet, Equal etc.)

Choose: natural sweeteners in limited amounts

1. Black Strap Molasses
2. Brown Rice syrup
3. Coconut palm sugar
4. Pure Maple Syrup
5. Raw Honey
6. Stevia
7. Sucanat
8. Xylitol

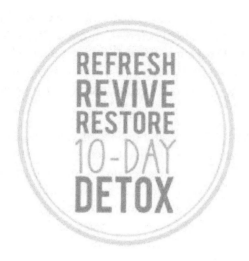

Superfood
Cheat Sheet

I encourage you to experiment with new, healthy foods you may not have tried before during your **Refresh Revive Restore 10-Day Detox**. You may find some ingredients that are new to you in the recipes or you may have heard about some of the super foods below and have wondered about their health benefits.

COCONUT OIL – is saturated fat but it is a medium-chain fatty acid which the body digests not as fat but rather as pure energy. Coconut oil will speed up your metabolism and also contains lauric acid which is anti-bacterial, anti-viral as well as an anti-fungal. It also improves adrenal and thyroid health. Coconut oil is a terrific choice for frying because it supports high heat.

RAW APPLE CIDER VINEGAR – Raw apple cider vinegar improves digestion, restores your body's natural pH and decreases inflammation. Consuming raw apple cider vinegar will increase your energy and improve liver function. It contains potassium, pectin, malic acid and calcium. Since it is not pasteurized, raw apple cider vinegar contains raw enzymes and gut-friendly bacteria which are good for your body.

RAW CACAO – The antioxidant benefits of raw cacao are amazing. It is also very high in magnesium, loaded with fiber and is a great source of natural iron.

FLAX SEEDS – Flax seeds are high in omega-3 fatty acids and rich in alpha linolenic acid (ALA). They also supply other nutrients such as manganese and magnesium as well as containing high amounts of fiber which aids in digestion.

CHIA SEEDS – Loaded with omega-3 fatty acids plus manganese, calcium and phosphorus- just one ounce of chia seeds contain 11 grams of fiber! This makes Chia seeds are wonderful for relieving constipation and improving heart health.

HEMP SEEDS – Hemp seeds contain all the omega fatty acids necessary for a healthy body. You only need 1 tablespoon per day to get your whole foods daily dose of omegas. They are also very high in protein.

SEA VEGETABLES – As a natural way to support the adrenals and the thyroid, sea vegetables are a wonderful addition. They are rich in minerals and trace elements including calcium, magnesium, iron, potassium, iodine, manganese and chromium.

Smoothie Boosters (also great in fresh pressed juices)

GINGER (in juice/smoothie) – Relieves motion sickness, nausea and morning sickness, stimulates circulation, soothing for colds and flus, relieves head and muscle aches, anti-inflammatory and fights infections.

TURMERIC (in juice/smoothie) – Anti-inflammatory, promotes liver function, supports cardiac health, alleviates nausea and soothes digestive complaints.

CHIA (in smoothie/juice) – Healthy gut function, antioxidant, supports tissue growth and repair, anti-inflammatory, supports heart health and lowers cholesterol.

MACA (in smoothie) – Boosts energy levels, immune support and balances hormones.

CACAO (in smoothie) – Antioxidant, releases endorphins, enhances mental alertness, supports blood vessel health and rich in magnesium.

FLAXSEED (in smoothie/juice) – Regulates bowel function, anti-inflammatory, supports heart health, promotes healthy tissue and detoxifies excess estrogen out of the body.

KEFIR (in smoothie/juice) – Probiotic, promotes healthy gut function, supports bone and teeth health as well as immune support.

WHEATGRASS (in juice/smoothie) –Anti-oxidant, anti-inflammatory, nourishes tissues, alkalizing and immune support.

PARSLEY (in juice/smoothie) – Relieves bloating and gas, stimulates digestive function, promotes thyroid, bladder and kidney health, anti-parasitic, anti-oxidant and alkalizing.

MINT (in juice/smoothie) – Relieves bloating and gas, soothes and relaxes digestive system, relieves pain, reduces nausea, clears nasal and chest congestion and boosts energy.

CINNAMON (in juice/smoothie) – Supports digestion, lessens nausea, stimulates circulation, antiviral, antifungal and balances blood sugar.

LEMON (in juice/smoothie) – Boosts immune function, fights colds and flus, antioxidant, antibacterial, promotes healthy tissue, supports liver detoxification and aids in gallbladder health.

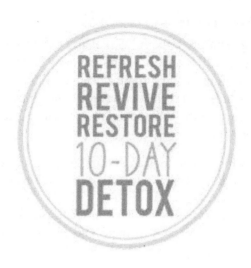

Detox Your Home

Detox Your Home

Reducing exposure to both internal and external toxins by detoxing your living space allows the body's own detoxification system to function more efficiently. This strengthens your resilience to the daily onslaught of factors which can impact your health. There many things that you can do to detox your home.

The following lists the most important steps that you can take to free your home from unnecessary chemical exposures:

- Avoid excess moisture accumulation as this encourages the growth of mold and mildew which can negatively impact health. Regularly monitor areas for moisture issues or leaks, particularly in basements. Clean surfaces where mold tends to grow around showers and tubs as well as beneath sinks.

- Avoid stain-guarded clothing, furniture and carpets due to the presence of PFC's (Per fluorinated compounds) which are cancer causing agents.

- Avoid wearing shoes in the house as most household dirt, pesticides and lead come in on your shoes. Go barefoot or wear slippers.

- Reduce toxins found in carpeting especially in products made from synthetic materials by using natural fiber wool and cotton rugs. Replace your carpeting with hardwood floors, all natural linoleum or ceramic tiles. Use nontoxic glues, adhesives, stains or sealers for installation.

- Receipts contain BPA which can leech onto your hands as well as on your produce. Do not leave your thermal receipts in your grocery bags.

- Contaminants in tap water become gases at room temperature. Install a shower filter to reduce the exposure to these toxins and this also prevents them from becoming airborne.

- Drinking water contains as many as 700 chemicals. Filter drinking water with a charcoal or reverse osmosis filter and avoid buying plastic BPA containing disposable water bottles.

- Regularly monitor carbon monoxide levels in your home. Leaks can occur through gas stoves, gas fireplaces, furnaces as well as chimneys and gas water heaters.

- House plants can help to detoxify the air in your home. The bacteria found in the soil can reduce the volatile organic compounds such as formaldehyde in the air.

- Indoor air is typically 2-5 times more polluted than outdoor air. Keep the air clean in your home by opening your windows and doors as much as possible to ventilate.

- Notice the recycling symbols on plastics and avoid numbers 1, 3 and 6 as well as clear plastics labelled number 7. This will cut down on your exposure to BPA, phthalates and styrene which are all highly toxic.

- Choose natural garden agents to replace toxic lawn and garden pesticides as well as herbicides.

- Do not use air fresheners or other synthetic fragrances. Choose natural essential oils to eliminate odor.

- Choose pure beeswax candles. Many other candles are petroleum-based which contain harmful chemicals such as benzene, toluene and ketones.

- Limit dry cleaning and remove or avoid the plastic wrap which traps the dry cleaning chemicals on clothes and in your closet. Let your dry cleaning air out, preferably outside, before storing it.

- When painting indoors, open all windows to ventilate properly. Choose less harmful, water based latex paint which contains low VOCs and has a low odor.

- Use a HEPA filter to vacuum your home which will reduce the levels of many chemicals. Vacuuming regularly will reduce your exposure to brominated fire retardants, phthalates and pesticides. Studies have identified 66 hormone-disrupting chemicals found in household dust.

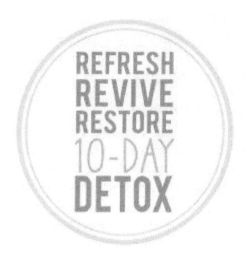

Detox Your Hormones

Detox Your Hormones

Many common household products contain harmful chemicals that can disrupt our hormones. These are commonly referred to as xenoestrogens.

What are Xenoestrogens?

In 1991, the field of xenoestrogens was first introduced to the world.[2] Xenoestrogens are foreign estrogens as "xeno" literally means foreign. Not found in nature, man-made toxins are estrogen imposters that make their way into the

body, pretending to be our own estrogen. They mimic the effects of the real hormone but over-stimulate cellular activity to an uncontrollable extent. Xenoestrogens are present in our soil, water, air and food supply as well as in personal care and household products. Xenoestrogens accumulate in the fat tissues of our bodies and have the capability of locking into our own estrogen's receptor sites. Xenoestrogens are highly toxic and harmful to our body and are one of the top causes of hormone imbalances!

Interesting Facts to Consider:

- By the time the average North American woman has completed her morning routine, she has exposed her face, body and hair to over **126 chemicals from 12 different products.**

---

[2] "Suite101: List of Xenoestrogens - Chemical Estrogens: How to Avoid Xenoestrogens," http://www.suite101.com/content/list-of-xenoestrogens---chemical-estrogens-a205523#ixzz1IrecjmqZ.

- According to the Environmental Protection Agency, 60% of what you put on your skin enters your blood stream and every organ in your body within **26 seconds**!

- The average North American contains **148 synthetic/toxic chemicals stored in the body.**

- Only **11% of the 10,500 chemicals** in cosmetics have been tested for safety!

- Xenoestrogens are **not found in nature** as they are man-made toxins that are estrogen imposters.

- **Xenoestrogens mimic the effects of the real hormone** but overstimulate cellular activity to an uncontrollable extent.

- **There are 70,000 registered chemicals** known as estrogen disruptors (xenoestrogens)!

How to Reduce Your Exposure to Xenoestrogens in Your Home

According to Environmental Defence, you should avoid the following **eleven toxic ingredients:**

1. 1,4-Dioxane
2. Artificial Musks
3. Coal Tar Derived Colours
4. BHA & BHT
5. 2 Formaldehyde Releasing Agents
6. Petroleum
7. Parabens
8. Phthalates
9. Silicone Chemicals

10. Triclosan
11. Bisphenol-A (BPA)

The Kitchen
The Pantry

- Avoid canned foods that are lined with plastic coating that contains Bisphenol-A (BPA)
- Avoid processed and packaged foods and choose packaged goods in glass or paper containers
- Purchase grains, nuts, dried fruits and beans in bulk and store in glass or stainless steel containers

Try these brands: San Remo Organics, Eat Wholesome Food Co., Amy's Organics, Pacific, Trader Joe's and Imagine

Side note- BPA- why you need to avoid it!

The Environment Defense recently set out to test 192 food cans that were collected from major retailers in North America and this is what they found:

- 17 of the 21 cans we tested contained BPA in the inner lining
- All three Canadian retailers included in this study sold food cans with BPA, including BPA in their private labels (President's Choice, No Name, Great Value, Compliments and Signal)
- All of Campbell's food cans tested contained BPA
- Broth and gravy cans were the most likely (100 per cent of tested cans overall) to contain BPA
- Cans of corn and peas were the least likely (41 per cent of tested cans overall) to contain BPA

- Many companies are replacing BPA-based resin with problematic types including polyvinyl chloride (or PVC which is a known carcinogen), polystyrene (a possible human carcinogen) and polyesters resins – all related to plastics

BPA was officially declared toxic in Canada in 2010 but it clearly still lurks in most of our canned food sources. BPA has been shown in repeated scientific studies to greatly increase the risk of breast and prostate cancers, infertility, early puberty in females, type 2 diabetes, obesity, asthma and impaired neurological development in children. **Purchase BPA free canned goods only**!

The Fridge

- Avoid all pesticides, herbicides and fungicides
- Choose organic, locally-grown and in-season foods
- Peel and thoroughly wash non-organic fruits and vegetables
- Buy hormone-free meats and dairy products to avoid hormones and pesticides

Try these brands: Organic food delivered right to your door- www.spud.ca; www.bluemoonorganics.com; www.chefsplate.com

Side note-the Dirty Dozen and Clean 15

The fruits and vegetables on "**The Dirty Dozen**" list when conventionally grown tested positive for at least 47 different chemicals with some testing positive for as many as 67. For produce on the "dirty" list, you should definitely **go organic**. "The Dirty Dozen" list includes:

1. Celery
2. Peaches
3. Strawberries
4. Apples
5. Domestic blueberries
6. Nectarines
7. Sweet bell peppers
8. Spinach, kale and collard greens
9. Cherries
10. Potatoes
11. Imported grapes
12. Lettuce

All the produce on "**The Clean 15**" bore little to no traces of pesticides and is safe to consume in non-organic form. This list includes:

1. Onions
2. Avocados
3. Sweet corn
4. Pineapples
5. Mango
6. Sweet peas
7. Asparagus
8. Kiwi fruit
9. Cabbage
10. Eggplant
11. Cantaloupe

12. Watermelon

13. Grapefruit

14. Sweet potatoes

15. Sweet onions

Cooking and Plastics

- Do not heat food in plastic containers
- Only use glass containers when heating foods
- Avoid Styrofoam containers as they contain BPA (drinking coffee out of a Styrofoam cup causes the BPA to leach out into the coffee)
- Avoid Teflon-coated nonstick pans which, if overheated, can release endocrine-disrupting compounds

Try these brands: Click here for the top 10 nonstick pans http://www.allcookwarefind.com/Non-Stick/

Food-Storage Containers

- Store your food in glass, ceramic or stainless steel food storage containers.
- Some plastic cling wrap is made from PVC (poly-vinyl chloride) which contains several types of xenoestrogens and other endocrine disruptors and should never touch food.
- Do not microwave food in plastic containers.
- Do not leave plastic containers, especially drinking water, in the sun.
- If a plastic water container has heated up significantly, throw it away.

- Do not refill plastic water bottles.
- Avoid freezing water in plastic bottles to drink later.

Try these brands: Click here for a variety of safer food and beverage storage options https://well.ca/categories/natural-food-drink-storage_2902.html   http://www.naturalathome.com/product-category/food-storage-containers

Click here for more information on water filtration systems https://wellnessmama.com/8079/water-filter-options/

Household Products

- Use chemical free, biodegradable laundry soap and avoid dryer sheets- try adding ½ cup of baking soda to the rinse cycle for softer laundry.
- Use chemical free household cleaning products.
- Choose chlorine-free products and unbleached paper products- toilet paper, paper towels and coffee filters.
- Use a chlorine filter on shower heads and filter drinking water.

Try these brands: Use this link to order Norwex cleaning products and partial proceeds go towards the Dr Cobi Scholarship fund to help those in need with health issues-http://sandraoben.norwex.biz/en_CA/customer/party/2009734 www.honest.com; www.seventhgeneration.com

Click here for Do It Yourself Recipes http://greatist.com/health/27-chemical-free-products-diy-spring-cleaning

Health and Beauty Products

Most people do not have the resources to replace all of their products at once. Start with the products that you use the most often. Examples include: moisturizer, sunscreen, mascara, soap, face wash, deodorant, makeup, lip products, shampoo, conditioner and toothpaste.

The following 3 tools will help you to determine if what you are using is toxic to your body:

1. Download and print the Environmental Defence's wallet-size green beauty guide. Check out the ingredients of your products to determine if they contain any of the top 10 body care toxins! http://environmentaldefence.ca/report/the-toxic-ten-pocket-guide/

2. Get the Environmental Working Group's (EWG) Skin Deep database app. This will help you to scan and search products for their toxicity ratings and find better alternatives. http://www.ewg.org/skindeep/

3. Download the Canadian app called Think Dirty Shop Clean. This app scans products and ranks them according to their toxic ingredients corresponding to their "dirty meter". It often provides a cleaner alternative as well. The products are ranked in the following scale:

   ✓ 3 or below is safe to use
   ✓ 4-6 need replacing with a better product once it runs out
   ✓ 7-10 needs immediate replacement (especially if pregnant)

   https://www.thinkdirtyapp.com/

Here are Tips to Get You Started:

- Avoid creams and cosmetics that have toxic chemicals and estrogenic ingredients such as parabens and stearalkonium chloride.
- Minimize your exposure to nail polish and nail polish removers.
- Use naturally based fragrances such as essential oils.
- Use chemical free soaps.
- Choose organic and natural feminine hygiene products.
- Choose natural toothpaste.
- Use chemical free Hair care products.

Try these Green Beauty Brands:

- I luv it Natural Deodorant http://www.iluvit.ca/
- Ela Spa http://www.ela-spa.com/
- 100% Pure https://ca.100percentpure.com/
- Clean Kiss Organics http://cleankissorganics.com/
- Ecco Bella Makeup http://www.eccobella.com/
- Pure and Simple https://pureandsimple.ca/
- Toothpaste- Kiss my Face http://kissmyface.com/;
- Jason's http://www.jason-personalcare.com/body-loving-products/oral ;
- Toms of Maine http://www.tomsofmaine.com/home

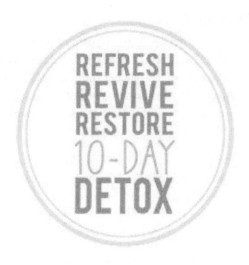

Detox Your Mind

Detox Your Mind

An emotional detox is just as important as detoxing your body and home. No amount of environmental toxins are as important as emotional toxicity. You can take many steps to clear toxins but if your house is full of anger, resentment, jealousy, unhappiness and a lack of love, compassion and forgiveness, the house will remain toxic!

It is estimated that up to 90% of illnesses are directly connected to our thought life. The average person has over 30,000 thoughts a day. Our thinking not only affects us emotionally but also physically. It is now realized that our thoughts can set the stage for sickness.

How can you tell if you need a mental detox? The following is a list of signs indicating that you need to detox your mind:

- Negative thought patterns
- Self-sabotaging actions
- Poor financial management
- Toxic relationships
- Outbursts of anger
- Easily irritated
- Relentless guilt
- Chronic stress
- Overspending
- Racing mind
- Conflict with others

If you have one or more of these signs, it is clear that you need to take action to detox your mind.

Detoxing your mind is an ongoing process that takes commitment and discipline. Determine your source of greatest toxicity and begin there. The following tips will help you to get started to detox your mind:

- Begin the day with a relaxation technique. Wake up a few minutes earlier, stay in bed and take 10 deep breaths, inhale and feel the peace enter your body and mind. Breathe in through your nose for the count of 4, hold for the count of 4 and breathe out through your mouth for the count of 4. Make sure that you are "belly breathing" and that your stomach is expanding as you inhale and not your chest.

- Every time you exhale, stress leaves your body. As you feel that peace, take it with you into the rest of your day. Whenever you feel stressed or anxious, bring those peaceful feelings back into your body and mind.

- Take control of your mental and emotional health by taking full responsibility for your thoughts, beliefs, responses and reactions. This is the first step in shifting to positive thinking.

- Detox your schedule! Assess your daily schedule and eliminate any unnecessary things that are causing stress, worry and rush!

- Quit tolerating the intolerable! Clean up your "outer house" (living environment) so that you can freely work on your "inner house" (your mind). Eliminate piles of clutter, unfinished projects and ask for what you need so that your home can be an uncluttered environment. Tolerations create stress, deplete your energy and steal your joy. Keep your home and environment clean, healthy, orderly and pleasing to your senses.

- Deal with stressful occurrences head on to prevent you from staying in a toxic thought cycle.

- Forgiveness is one of the most important ways to detox your mind. Holding on to resentment and bitterness poisons your mind, body and spirit. It is essential to let the past go. Forgiveness literally means giving up the hope of a better past.

- Avoid mental and physical toxins whenever possible. Fill your mind and spirit with positive and nurturing thoughts.

- Take a Technology Break. Make it a low-tech day. Keep your television, computer, cellphone and other electronics turned off for at least one day a week as well as in the evenings.

- Schedule some time for yourself. Set aside some time each week to have a night out with a partner, a night in on your own or some time out with friends. Give yourself an opportunity to relax and have fun as you leave all your other stresses behind. Having something to look forward to is an essential part of living a balanced life.

- Focus on the purpose for your life. What is the main passion in your life? Is it to be excellent in your job, have your own business, be an incredible parent or to master a skill or a hobby? Discover the purpose for your life and write a list of all the things you need to do in order to live a purpose filled life.

- Work toward your purpose on a daily basis. So often we can feel that we are getting stressed, busy and anxious and then we lose sight of our unique purpose. If you have an overall vision for your life that you are working toward, it will bring a sense of peace and calm to your mind.

- Hydration is essential to a healthy mind. Recent studies have revealed that even mild dehydration can alter a person's mood, energy level and ability to think clearly. Approximately 2/3 of your body is water. You need to keep it hydrated throughout the day in order for it to work properly.

- Live your life with awe, wonder and passion. Turn situations around by refusing to allow any negativity which can hamper the incredible life that you have chosen to live.

Make these tips to detox your mind a priority. Your life will turn around and you will start to enjoy living a purpose filled life.

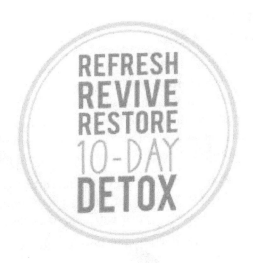

Let's Get Started!

Where to Start?

Eliminate the "bad guys"

In order to detoxify effectively, we need to eliminate the foods that are compromising our system. Every minute of every day, our body is dealing with foreign invaders. These toxins come from the air we breathe to the foods we eat and drink as well as exposure to the chemicals found in our homes, cleaning supplies, body care products and more.

By starting with the elimination of the foods that cause the most stress in our systems, we can then begin to eliminate the toxic buildup and create an environment for our cells to thrive!

Foods to **AVOID** during the **Refresh Revive Restore 10-Day Detox:**

- ✓ **ALL GLUTEN** – pasta, bread, cereal, baked goods, crackers and whole wheat products
- ✓ **ALL DAIRY** – milk, ice cream, cheese, yogurt and cream
- ✓ **ALL SUGAR** – all processed sugars (see 10-Day Kitchen Clean Out Guide for safe choices in limited amounts)
- ✓ **ALL PROCESSED FOODS** – canned/boxed foods
- ✓ **ALL ALCOHOL**
- ✓ **CAFFEINE** – coffee and black tea
- ✓ **HIGH FAT FOODS** – anything that is deep fried
- ✓ **RED MEAT** – unless it is grass-fed, hormone and antibiotic free beef

Refer to the Kitchen Clean Out Cheat Sheet for more information about what to keep and what to toss from your kitchen.

3-Day Refresh Revive Restore Liquid Cleanse

Here is how it works:

- During the entire duration of the **Refresh Revive Restore 10-Day Detox,** you will consume 1 large glass of warm water with the juice of ½ a squeezed lemon every morning before consuming anything else.
- During the first 3 days, enjoy 3 "liquid" meals per day.
- Breakfast and lunch will be a protein rich green smoothie.
- Dinner will consist of a pureed soup.
- Consume 3L of water a day (feel free to flavor with fresh fruit or veggies).
- Green tea and other herbal teas are allowed.
- Take your suggested supplements (if you are taking prescribed medications, make sure to consult your pharmacist or medical doctor).
- Refer to the snack chart if you need to eat something extra in between meals.
- **Note:** If the 3-day liquid cleanse is not an option for you, then follow the instructions for the remaining 7 days but over a 10-day period.

3-Day Body Reset Detox Liquid Cleanse

Day 1

Note: 1-2 snacks can be consumed as needed during the 3-Day Liquid Cleanse.

BREAKFAST	LUNCH	DINNER
Kale Avocado Smoothie	*Emerald Smoothie*	*Butternut Squash Soup*
2 cups chopped kale Half an avocado 1 cup fresh or frozen berries 1 tbsp. chia seeds 1 scoop vegan vanilla protein *(See 10-Day Detox Supplement Guide for the Top Vegan Protein Powders)* 1 cup unsweetened almond/coconut/cashew milk 1 cup water Blend & enjoy!	Half a cucumber, chopped 1 cup chopped spinach Half an apple, chopped 1 cup romaine, chopped Juice of half a lemon 1 tbsp. grated fresh ginger 1 scoop vegan vanilla protein *(See 10-Day Detox Supplement Guide for the Top Vegan Protein Powders)* 1-2 cups water Blend & enjoy!	1 large butternut squash, peeled & chopped into chunks 1 large onion, chopped 3 garlic cloves, chopped 2 tbsp. curry powder (use less or more, depending on preference) 1 tsp. ground cinnamon ½ tsp. ground nutmeg 1 tbsp. coconut oil Vegetable broth and/or water Sea salt and pepper Walnuts, chopped-for garnish (optional) *refer to full recipe in recipe section*

Day 2

BREAKFAST	LUNCH	DINNER
Clean & Green Smoothie	*Berry Almond Butter Smoothie*	*Sweet Potato Soup*
2 cups kale, chopped 2-3 celery stalks, chopped Half a cucumber, chopped 2 tbsp. cilantro, chopped (optional) 1 apple, chopped Half a banana, chopped 1 scoop vegan vanilla protein *(See 10-Day Detox Supplement Guide for the Top Vegan Protein Powders)* Juice of half a lemon Enough water to blend thoroughly – approx. 1-2 cups Blend & Enjoy!	½ cup blueberries 1 tbsp. almond butter 1 tbsp. chia seeds 1 scoop vegan vanilla protein *(See 10-Day Detox Supplement Guide for the Top Vegan Protein Powders)* 1 cup unsweetened almond/coconut/cashew milk 1 cup water Blend & Enjoy!	2 tbsp. olive oil 2 onions, peeled and chopped 2 carrots, peeled and chopped 2 celery stalks, chopped 1 large sweet potato, cut into small chunks 2-3 cups chicken broth 1 tsp. cinnamon Sea salt and freshly ground black pepper, to taste *refer to full recipe in recipe section*

Day 3

BREAKFAST	LUNCH	DINNER
Choose Day 1 or Day 2 Smoothie	*Choose Day 1 or Day 2 Smoothie*	*Consume leftover Butternut Squash or Sweet Potato Soup*

Refresh Revive Restore
10-Day Detox
3-Day Liquid Cleanse Soup Recipes

Butternut Squash Soup
Ingredients

- ✓ 1 large butternut squash, peeled and chopped into chunks
- ✓ 1 large onion, chopped
- ✓ 3 garlic cloves, chopped
- ✓ 2 tbsp. curry powder (use less or more, depending on preference)
- ✓ 1 tsp. ground cinnamon
- ✓ ½ tsp. ground nutmeg
- ✓ 1 tbsp. coconut oil
- ✓ 3-4 cups vegetable broth and/or water to cover squash
- ✓ Sea salt and freshly ground black pepper, to taste
- ✓ 8 walnuts, chopped, for garnish (optional)

Directions

1. In a large pot, sauté onion in coconut oil for a few minutes. Once onion has softened, add garlic, spices, salt, pepper and stir. Sauté for 1 minute.

2. Add butternut squash and cover with vegetable broth or water. Add just enough liquid to cover the squash. Cook on medium-low heat for 15-20 minutes or until squash is soft and cooked through.

3. Transfer to a blender and puree soup. Transfer back to pot and adjust spices to taste as necessary.

4. Serve hot with a tbsp. of chopped walnuts and a sprinkle of cinnamon.

Sweet Potato Soup
Ingredients

- ✓ 2 tbsp. extra virgin olive oil
- ✓ 2 onions, peeled and chopped
- ✓ 2 carrots, peeled and chopped
- ✓ 2 celery stalks, chopped
- ✓ 1 large sweet potato or 2 small, peeled and cut into small chunks
- ✓ 2-3 cups vegetable broth
- ✓ 1 tsp. cinnamon
- ✓ Sea salt and freshly ground black pepper, to taste

Directions

1. In a large saucepan or soup pot sauté onions, carrots and celery over medium heat in olive oil.

2. Add the sweet potatoes and enough broth to completely cover all the vegetables.

3. Season with cinnamon, salt and pepper and bring to a simmer.

4. Cook until potatoes are very soft and then puree with a hand blender, food processor or countertop blender until smooth.

5. Adjust spices as needed for taste.

Refresh Revive Restore
10-Day Detox Snacks

It is common to get hungry in between meals. Feel free to make another Clean & Green smoothie to drink between meals or choose from the following:

- ✓ 10 almonds
- ✓ 5 macadamia nuts
- ✓ 1 small apple with 1 tbsp. almond butter/cashew butter/hemp seed butter
- ✓ 1-2 cups celery sticks/sliced peppers/cucumbers/carrots with 2 tbsp. organic hummus

NOTE: Do not have the same snack twice in one day as variety is important

Or choose the snack salad option:

Mixed Green Salad
Ingredients

- ✓ 1 large handful of mixed organic greens
- ✓ Half a cucumber, chopped
- ✓ 3-4 cherry tomatoes, chopped
- ✓ Finely chopped red onion
- ✓ 1 tbsp. hemp seeds

Salad Dressing
Ingredients

- ✓ 2 tbsp. extra virgin olive oil

✓ 2 tsp. balsamic vinegar

✓ Juice of half a lemon

✓ 1 tsp. dried oregano

✓ 1 garlic clove, crushed

Directions

1. Mix all ingredients together and pour over salad.
- Continue to start the day with 1/2 lemon squeezed into 1 cup of warm water.

Refresh Revive Restore 10-Day Detox 7-Day Meal Plan (after the 3-Day Liquid Cleanse)

- Chose to follow either the **vegan/vegetarian or protein meal plan** (or combine meals between the two) for the 7 days after the 3-Day Liquid Cleanse is complete.
- You can continue enjoying your morning green smoothie for breakfast or choose an option for breakfast from the meal plan.
- If you are hungry between meals, choose a snack from the snack list or the snack salad option.
- Continue to avoid all of the foods listed on page 5.
- Continue to drink 3L of water a day (drink in between meals).
- Make an effort to get a minimum of 7 hours minimum of sleep per night.
- Walk for at least 30 minutes per day.

7 Day Meal Plan Vegan/Vegetarian

Note: These meal plans are suggestions. Feel free to mix things up as long as you follow the recommended guidelines. Make extra dinner and bring leftovers for lunch the next day. Make a double batch of any recipe and freeze for later. Keep breakfast quick and easy and continue to have one of the smoothies from the first 3 days of the detox.

VEGETARIAN

	BREAKFAST	LUNCH	DINNER
Day 1	Chocolate Raspberry Smoothie	Best Ever Red Lentil Dahl	Green Goodness Bowl
Day 2	Chocolate Hazelnut Protein Bowl	Sweet Potato and Black Bean Salad	Moroccan Chickpea Soup
Day 3	Energizing Blueberry Spinach Smoothie	Avocado Tomato Quinoa Salad	Spicy Sesame Tofu with Quinoa Pilaf
Day 4	Coco-no-Oat Granola	Grilled Chickpea Stuffed Avocados	Roasted Veggies with Tempeh, Quinoa and Dried Cranberries
Day 5	Vanilla Maple Chia Pudding	Kale Caesar Salad and Broccoli Avocado Soup	Butternut Squash and Pesto Pizza
Day 6	Sweet Green Morning Smoothie	Spinach Lentil Soup	Happy Vegan Bowl
Day 7	Acai Breakfast Bowl	Apple Quinoa Salad	The Best Tempeh Vegan Chili

7 Day Meal Plan Protein

Note- These meal plans are suggestions. Feel free to mix things up as long as you follow the recommended guidelines. Make extra dinner and bring leftovers for lunch the next day. Make a double batch of any recipe and freeze for later. Keep breakfast quick and easy and continue to have one of the smoothies from the first 3 days of the detox. Cook 4 chicken breasts at a time to have some on hand.

PROTEIN

	BREAKFAST	LUNCH	DINNER
Day 1	Turkey Veggie Frittata	Green Goodness Bowl with Chicken	Garlic Chili Shrimp with Pesto Zoodles
Day 2	Protein Packed Gluten Free Crepes	Rainbow Collard Wraps	Cauliflower Fried Rice
Day 3	Chocolate Hazelnut Protein Power Bowl	Tuna Toss Up	Roasted Lemon Rosemary Chicken
Day 4	Energizing Blueberry Spinach Smoothie	Detox Green Salad with Pumpkin Seeds and Chicken	Meatloaf Muffins
Day 5	Veggie Egg Muffins	Kale Salad with Meatloaf Muffins	Spaghetti Squash Bake with Italian Sausage and Herbs

| Day 6 | Coco-no-Oat Granola | Green Egg White Scramble | Slow Cooker Whole Roasted Chicken |
| Day 7 | Vanilla Maple Chia Pudding | Apple Quinoa Salad | Coconut Ginger Salmon with Roasted Asparagus |

Refresh Revive Restore 10-Day Detox Supplements

Suggestions. If you are taking any prescription medications, you should discuss adding in supplements with your pharmacist and/or medical doctor prior to taking anything new.

Refer to the **Refresh Revive Restore 10-Day Detox Supplement Guide** for more information and brand suggestions.

Recommended Supplements:

- ✓ Greens Powder
- ✓ Probiotics
- ✓ Digestive Enzymes
- ✓ Liver Support and Detoxification
- ✓ Vegan Protein Powder

Refresh Revive Restore 10-Day Detox Tips for Success

- ✓ Be gentle with yourself. Your body is not used to eating this way so it is important to shop, prepare and plan ahead so that you are not unprepared at meal time.

✓ Let your family and friends know that you are treating yourself to a **Refresh Revive Restore 10-Day Detox** and will be making some changes in your nutrition and lifestyle for the next 10 days (and hopefully longer). Ask them to join you!

✓ Include walking a minimum of 30 minutes per day during the **Refresh Revive Restore 10-Day Detox** at a minimum. Enjoy your regular exercise routine during the detox and after. Sweating helps to release toxins and improve the lymphatic system which allows for greater detoxification.

✓ You many experience light-headedness, headaches or feel fatigued during your 3-Day Liquid Cleanse. This is normal as your body is releasing toxins. Listen to your body and rest as required. Consume 1-2 extra snacks if needed to keep your blood sugar levels stabilized.

✓ Always carry snacks with you. Feeling hunger is normal and indicates that your stomach capacity is shrinking and this is positive. Avoid feeling extreme or uncomfortable hunger.

✓ Enjoy a nightly Epsom salt bath: 2 cups Epsom salts in hot water. Submerge as much of your body as you can. Relax for 20-30 minutes. When you get out, do not towel dry. Wrap yourself in a big towel and lay down for 30 minutes. This will allow your body to further detoxify through sweating.

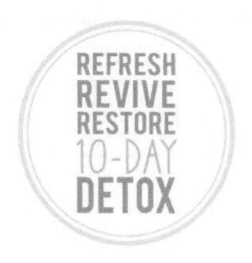

Recharge and Energize Your Body!

7 Day Meal Plan Recipes

7 Day Meal Plan Vegan/Vegetarian

Note- These meal plans are suggestions. Feel free to mix things up as long as you follow the recommended guidelines. Make extra dinner and bring leftovers for lunch the next day. Make a double batch of any recipe and freeze for later. Keep breakfast quick and easy and continue to have one of the smoothies from the first 3 days of the detox.

VEGETARIAN

	BREAKFAST	LUNCH	DINNER
Day 1	Chocolate Raspberry Smoothie	Best Ever Red Lentil Dahl	Green Goodness Bowl
Day 2	Chocolate Hazelnut Protein Bowl	Sweet Potato and Black Bean Salad	Moroccan Chickpea Soup
Day 3	Energizing Blueberry Spinach Smoothie	Avocado Tomato Quinoa Salad	Spicy Sesame Tofu with Quinoa Pilaf
Day 4	Coco-no-Oat Granola	Grilled Chickpea Stuffed Avocados	Roasted Veggies with Tempeh, Quinoa and Dried Cranberries
Day 5	Vanilla Maple Chia Pudding	Kale Caesar Salad and Broccoli Avocado Soup	Butternut Squash and Pesto Pizza
Day 6	Sweet Green Morning Smoothie	Spinach Lentil Soup	Happy Vegan Bowl
Day 7	Acai Breakfast Bowl	Apple Quinoa Salad	The Best Tempeh Vegan Chili

7 Day Meal Plan Protein

Note- These meal plans are suggestions. Feel free to mix things up as long as you follow the recommended guidelines. Make extra dinner and bring leftovers for lunch the next day. Make a double batch of any recipe and freeze for later. Keep breakfast quick and easy and continue to have one of the smoothies from the first 3 days of the detox. Cook 4 chicken breasts at a time to have some on hand.

PROTEIN

	BREAKFAST	LUNCH	DINNER
Day 1	Turkey Veggie Frittata	Green Goodness Bowl with Chicken	Garlic Chili Shrimp with Pesto Zoodles
Day 2	Protein Packed Gluten Free Crepes	Rainbow Collard Wraps	Cauliflower Fried Rice
Day 3	Chocolate Hazelnut Protein Power Bowl	Tuna Toss Up	Roasted Lemon Rosemary Chicken
Day 4	Energizing Blueberry Spinach Smoothie	Detox Green Salad with Pumpkin Seeds and Chicken	Meatloaf Muffins
Day 5	Veggie Egg Muffins	Kale Salad with Meatloaf Muffins	Spaghetti Squash Bake with Italian Sausage and Herbs

Day 6	Coco-no-Oat Granola	Green Egg White Scramble	Slow Cooker Whole Roasted Chicken
Day 7	Vanilla Maple Chia Pudding	Apple Quinoa Salad	Coconut Ginger Salmon with Roasted Asparagus

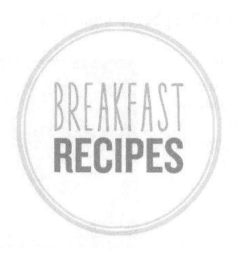

Vegan/Vegetarian
Meal Plan Recipes

Chocolate Raspberry Smoothie

Ingredients

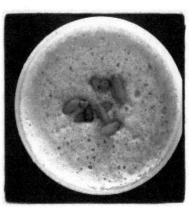

- 1 scoop vanilla vegan protein powder
- 1/3 cup frozen raspberries
- 1 Tbsp. almond butter
- 2 tsp. chia seeds
- 1 tsp. cinnamon
- 1 Tbsp. raw cacao powder
- 2 cups unsweetened almond milk (or non-dairy milk of choice)
- Goji berries for topping (optional)

Instructions

1. Add all ingredients into blender, blend and enjoy!

Chocolate Hazelnut Protein Bowl

Ingredients

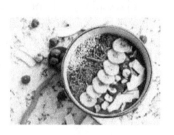

- 1 frozen banana
- ¼ cup hazelnuts, soaked 30 minutes
- 3 Tbsp. hemp seeds
- 2 Tbsp. raw cacao powder
- 1 scoop chocolate protein powder
- ¾ cup coconut milk
- 1 tsp. cinnamon
- ice (optional)
- 1/4 avocado (optional and may be needed for additional thickness and consistency)

Optional Toppings

- Strawberries
- Cacao nibs
- Shredded coconut
- Hemp seeds
- Chia seeds
- Goji berries
- Hazelnuts
- Sesame Seeds
- Pumpkins Seeds

Instructions

1. Place all ingredients (minus the toppings) into a blender and blend until well combined. Pour into a bowl and top with your favourite ingredients.

2. Topping with hemp seeds, chia seeds and other superfoods will give this bowl a super antioxidant kick and supply you with an abundance of plant based protein and healthy fats.

Energizing Blueberry Spinach Smoothie

Ingredients

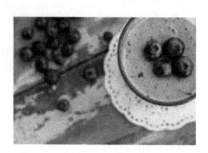

- 1/2 cup frozen blueberries
- 1/4 avocado
- 2 large handfuls of organic spinach
- 2 cups water coconut water
- 1 cup almond milk
- 1 scoop vanilla vegan protein powder
- 1 Tbsp. chia seeds
- 3-4 ice cubes (optional)
- 1 tsp. cinnamon

Instructions

1. Blend together in a high speed blender.

Coco-No-Oat Granola

Ingredients

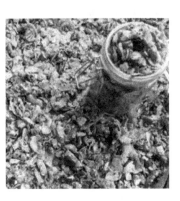

- 3 cups coconut flakes, unsweetened
- 1 cup pecans, roughly chopped
- ½ cup pumpkin seeds
- ½ cup almonds, roughly chopped
- 2 Tbsp. chia seeds
- 2 tsp. cinnamon
- 5-6 Tbsp. coconut oil, melted
- 2 tsp. maple syrup

Instructions

1. Preheat oven to 250°F and line a baking sheet with parchment paper.
2. Combine all ingredients in a large bowl, then spread evenly on a tray. (You could use 2 trays or 1 large one).
3. Bake for 20-30 minutes, until golden and desired crispness is reached.
4. Be sure to remove from the oven halfway and gently stir.

Vanilla Maple Chia Pudding

Ingredients

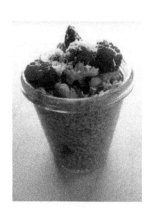

- 3/4 cup chia seeds
- 4 cups unsweetened almond or coconut milk
- 1/2 tsp. ground vanilla bean
- 1 tsp. cinnamon
- 2 tsp. maple syrup
- Pinch of Himalayan sea salt

Instructions

1. In a large mason jar, add all your ingredients.
2. Secure jar with lid and give it a good shake. Alternatively, you can add everything to a blender and blend together for a few seconds, then pour into your mason jar.
3. Leave in fridge overnight.
4. In the morning, shake again really well, then pour out desired serving into a bowl.
5. Top with your favourite superfood ingredients!

Notes:

- I topped mine with fresh picked organic raspberries, chopped walnuts and shredded coconut.
- This also makes a great healthy dessert! Add a Tbsp. of raw cacao powder to the mix for a chocolatey boost!

Sweet Green Morning Smoothie

Ingredients

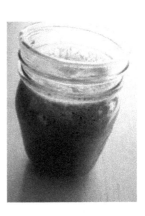

- 2 cups water or coconut water
- 1 pear or 1/2 cup fresh chopped pineapple
- Large handful of kale, washed and de-stemmed
- Large handful of spinach, washed
- 1 Tbsp. hemp seeds
- 1 tsp. chia seeds
- 1 scoop vanilla vegan protein powder
- 1 tsp. cinnamon

Instructions

1. Add all ingredients into blender and blend on high until well combined.
2. Drink and enjoy.

Acai Breakfast Bowl

Ingredients

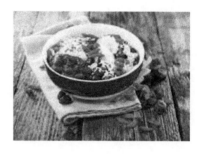

- ¼ cup unsweetened almond or coconut milk
- 1 package (100g) of frozen acai (I use Sambazon unsweetened pure acai)
- 1 cup frozen berries (raspberries, blueberries, strawberries, blackberries)
- 1 scoop vanilla vegan protein powder
- ¼ cup gluten free granola (optional)
- ¼ cup sliced banana (optional)
- 1/3 cup of your favorite mixed Superfoods (optional)

Instructions

1. Break the frozen acai up into large chunks while still in the package.
2. Remove from packaging and place frozen acai, frozen berries, milk and protein powder, if using, into blender.
3. Transfer mixture into a bowl and top with your favourite ingredients.

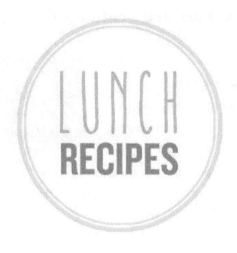

Vegan/Vegetarian
Meal Plan Recipes

The Best Ever Red Lentil Dahl

Ingredients

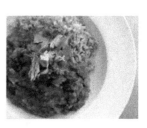

- 2 Tbsp. coconut oil
- 1 medium onion, chopped
- 3 large garlic cloves, minced
- 2 Tbsp. freshly grated ginger
- 2-3 large carrots, peeled and finely diced
- 2 tsp. curry powder (or more to taste, based on preference)
- 1 tsp. ground cumin
- 1/2 tsp. ground turmeric
- 1 1/2 cups dried red lentils, rinsed and picked through
- 1 (14-oz) can of light coconut milk
- 2 cups low-sodium vegetable broth
- 1/2 tsp. Sea salt and fresh cracked pepper
- 1 (5 oz.) package of baby spinach
- 2 cups cooked brown rice or quinoa (optional)
- Cilantro and green onion for garnish (optional)

Instructions

1. Pour oil into a large pot over medium heat. Add in chopped onion, garlic and a pinch of salt. Stir to combine. Sauté over medium heat for 4-5 minutes, stirring occasionally, until onions have softened.

2. Stir in the ginger and the carrots and continue sautéing for 3-4 more minutes.

3. Add in the curry powder, cumin and turmeric. Stir well. Cook for a minute, until fragrant.

4. Stir in entire can of coconut milk, red lentils, broth and salt. Bring to a simmer and reduce heat to medium-low. Cook, covered with the lid ajar, for roughly 15-20 minutes or until the lentils and carrots are tender. Stir occasionally to prevent the lentils from sticking. Add a touch more broth if you prefer a thinner consistency.

5. Once lentils are cooked, turn off the heat and stir in the spinach. Combine it with the dahl and the heat will help to wilt the spinach.

6. Serve over basmati rice or quinoa and garnish with cilantro and green onions.

7. This dahl will keep for up to a week in the fridge or 4-5 weeks frozen and can be enjoyed throughout the winter.

Sweet Potato and Black Bean Salad

Ingredients

- 2 sweet potatoes, diced and cut into ½ inch chunks
- 1 Tbsp. extra virgin olive oil
- 1 tsp. cumin
- ½ tsp. cinnamon
- ½ tsp. paprika
- 4 Tbsp. tahini
- ½ lemon, juiced
- 2 garlic cloves, minced
- 1/8 cup unsweetened almond milk
- 1 can black beans, drained and rinsed
- 2 cups cherry tomatoes, halved
- Sea salt and black pepper, to taste
- 1 cup fresh parsley, chopped

Instructions

1. Preheat the oven to 400°F.
2. Line a large baking sheet with parchment paper.
3. In a large mixing bowl, combine diced sweet potato, olive oil, cumin, cinnamon and paprika. Transfer to baking sheet and bake for 25 minutes.
4. Meanwhile, make your tahini dressing by whisking together tahini, lemon juice, minced garlic and almond milk.

Avocado Tomato Quinoa Salad

Ingredients

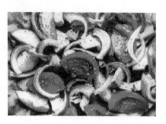

- 1 avocado, chopped
- 2 cups cooked quinoa
- 1 cup cherry tomatoes, chopped
- 1 cup cucumbers, chopped
- 1 Tbsp. red onion, chopped

Dressing

- 1 Tbsp. extra virgin olive oil
- 2 tsp. balsamic dressing
- Juice of half a lemon
- Pinch of sea salt

Instructions

1. Mix all ingredients together in a salad bowl and enjoy!

Grilled Chickpea Stuffed Avocados

Ingredients

- 1/2 cup frozen peas, thawed
- 1/2 cup organic frozen corn, thawed
- 1/2 cup cherry tomatoes, halved
- 1 Lemon, juiced
- 2 Tbsp. Tahini
- 1 can Chickpeas, drained and rinsed
- 1 Tbsp. extra virgin olive oil
- 1 Tbsp. Chili powder
- Sea salt & black pepper, to taste
- 2 avocados, halved and pits removed
- 1/4 cup parsley, chopped

Instructions

1. Preheat grill to medium heat.
2. Combine the peas, corn and cherry tomatoes in a bowl. Set aside.
3. Combine the lemon and tahini together in a small jar. Seal and shake well. Set aside. (Tip: Add extra water, 1 Tbsp. at a time if the dressing is too thick.)
4. In a small bowl, toss your chickpeas with olive oil and chili powder. Season with sea salt and black pepper to taste. Toss well until coated and transfer into a grilling basket. Grill for 15 - 20 minutes or until crispy. Toss with tongs periodically to prevent burning.

5. Brush the flesh of the avocado with a bit of olive oil then place face down on the grill. Grill for 5 minutes.

6. Remove the avocados from the grill. Stuff with the peas, corn and tomato mix. Add chickpeas on top, then drizzle with tahini sauce. Garnish with chopped parsley and enjoy!

Kale Caesar Salad

Salad Ingredients

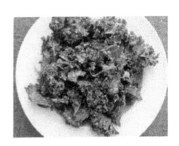

- 5-6 cups (1 large bunch) raw kale, massaged
- 2 Tbsp. hemp seeds
- 1 Tbsp. nutritional yeast

Caesar Dressing Ingredients

- ½ cup raw cashews, soaked overnight or for 4 hours
- 1 Tbsp. tahini
- 1 cup water
- 3 Tbsp. nutritional yeast
- Juice of 1 large lemon
- 3 garlic cloves
- 2 tsp. Dijon mustard
- Sea salt and black pepper to taste

Instructions

1. Massage kale to soften in a large salad bowl and set aside.
2. Add all Caesar dressing ingredients into a food processor and blend until well combined. You may need to add more water, depending on the consistency you like.
3. Add dressing to salad and top with hemp seeds and nutritional yeast.

Broccoli Avocado Soup

Ingredients

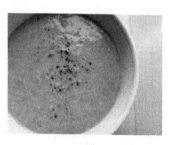

- 1 Tbsp. coconut oil
- 1 medium yellow onion, diced
- 3 cloves garlic, minced
- 1/4 tsp. red pepper flakes
- 4-6 cups vegetable broth (enough to cover the broccoli)
- 1 head broccoli, trimmed and chopped (about 6 cups)
- 2 cups baby spinach
- 1 avocado, chopped
- Sea salt and freshly ground black pepper

Instructions

1. Heat oil in a medium pot over medium heat. Add onion, garlic and pepper flakes and cook, stirring, until tender, 6 to 8 minutes. Add broth and bring to a boil. Add broccoli and cook, covered, until bright green and tender, about 3-5 minutes.
2. Season with salt and pepper.
3. Remove from heat and stir in spinach.
4. Transfer soup to a blender and purée with avocado.
5. Adjust seasonings and garnish with fresh pepper.

Spinach Lentil Soup

Ingredients

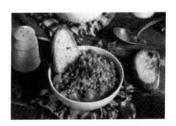

- 1 Tbsp. extra-virgin olive oil
- 1 medium celery stalk, diced
- 1 medium carrot, peeled and diced
- 1/2 medium yellow onion, diced
- 3 medium garlic cloves, minced
- Sea salt and ground black pepper
- 1 quart low-sodium vegetable broth
- 1 (15-ounce) can diced tomatoes with their juices
- 1 1/4 cups green lentils (any colour will do except red), rinsed
- 1 bay leaf
- 1/4 tsp. finely chopped fresh thyme leaves
- 1/2 tsp. dried oregano
- 1 tsp. red wine vinegar or balsamic vinegar
- 1 large bunch spinach leaves

Instructions

1. Heat the oil in a large saucepan over medium heat. Add the celery, carrot and onion-cook, stirring occasionally until the vegetables have softened, about 10 minutes.

2. Stir in the garlic and cook until fragrant, about 1 minute.

3. Season with several generous pinches of salt and pepper.

4. Add the broth, tomatoes with their juices, lentils, bay leaf, thyme and oregano, stir to combine. Cover and bring to a simmer, about 15 minutes.

5. Once simmering, reduce the heat to low and continue simmering, covered, until the lentils and vegetables are soft, about 15 minutes more.

6. Taste and season with more salt or pepper as needed, then stir in the vinegar.

7. Add the spinach and stir until wilted. If you prefer a creamier texture, purée half of the soup in a blender or with a hand blender. Enjoy!

Apple Quinoa Salad

Ingredients

- 1 cup cooked quinoa
- 1/2 cup chopped walnuts
- 1/2 small red bell pepper, chopped
- 1/3 cup red onion, chopped
- 1/2 cup fresh parsley, chopped
- 1/4 cup lemon juice
- 2 -3 Tbsp. vegetable broth
- Salt and pepper to taste
- 1/4 tsp. cinnamon
- 1 clove minced garlic
- 1 large chopped apple

Instructions

1. Make sure the quinoa is cooled before starting this recipe.
2. Mix all ingredients except for the quinoa, walnuts and apple.
3. Once combined, add the quinoa, walnuts and apple and mix well.

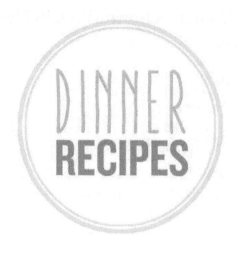

Vegan/Vegetarian Meal Plan Recipes

Green Goodness Bowl with Dill Hummus Dressing

Ingredients

- ½ cup hummus
- ½ lemon, juiced
- 1 Tbsp. Extra virgin olive oil
- ½ cup fresh dill
- Sea salt and black pepper (to taste)
- 1 Tbsp. coconut oil
- 8 cups Kale leaves
- 1 zucchini, diced
- 1 cup frozen edamame, thawed
- 1 cup frozen peas, thawed
- ½ cup raw cashews
- 1 Avocado, sliced
- 4 green onions, chopped

Instructions

1. In a jar, combine hummus, lemon juice, olive oil and dill-season with sea salt and black pepper. Shake well and set aside. You may need to add 1 Tbsp. of warm water to thin depending on the consistency of your hummus.

2. Heat coconut oil in a large pan over medium heat. Add kale, zucchini and sauté until kale is just wilted. Remove from heat and set aside.

3. Divide kale and zucchini between bowls and top with edamame, green peas, green onions, cashews and avocado. Drizzle with dill hummus dressing.

Moroccan Chickpea Soup

Ingredients

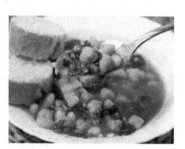

- 1 large onion, medium diced
- 5 to 6 garlic cloves, finely chopped
- 1 tsp. ground cinnamon
- 1 tsp. ground cumin
- 1/8 tsp. cayenne pepper
- 1 heaping tsp. sweet or smoked paprika
- 1 (14.5-ounce) can organic chopped tomatoes
- 2 (398ml) cans organic chickpeas, drained and rinsed well
- 1-quart organic low sodium vegetable broth
- 1 tsp. coconut sugar
- 1 Tbsp. extra virgin olive oil
- Sea salt and ground black pepper
- 1 (5-ounce) package pre-washed organic baby spinach

Instructions

1. Heat extra virgin olive oil in a large pot over medium-high heat. Add onion and garlic- sauté until the onions begin to turn translucent and lower heat if browning starts to occur.

2. Add spices and sauté a minute or so.

3. Add tomatoes, chickpeas, broth and sugar. Season with a couple pinches of salt and 10 grinds of fresh pepper. Stir well.

4. Chickpeas should be just covered with liquid. If level is shy, add some water so the chickpeas are just covered.

5. Bring to a simmer, then lower heat and gently simmer for 35-40 minutes.

6. Remove soup from heat. Use a potato masher to mash up some of the chickpeas in the pot.

7. Stir in the spinach and let the heat through until wilted, just a couple of minutes.

8. Season with salt and pepper to taste.

9. Serve soup hot and drizzle lightly with extra virgin olive oil, if desired.

10. Enjoy!

Spicy Sesame Tofu with Quinoa Pilaf

Ingredients

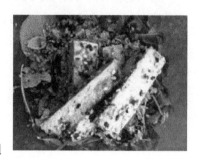

- 14 ounces' extra-firm organic tofu
- 1/4 cup maple syrup
- 3 Tbsp. gluten free tamari
- 3 Tbsp. finely chopped fresh ginger
- 2 Tbsp. sesame oil
- 2 Tbsp. rice vinegar or apple cider vinegar
- 2 cloves of finely chopped garlic
- 1 tsp. red pepper flakes
- 1 Tbsp. extra virgin olive oil
- 1/4 cup mixed white and black sesame seeds, lightly toasted
- Pinch of cayenne pepper

Instructions

1. Rinse tofu under cold water, press out liquid and set aside.
2. Meanwhile, mix maple syrup, tamari, ginger, sesame oil, vinegar, garlic and chili flakes into a small saucepan and bring just to a simmer. Keep warm.
3. Cut tofu lengthwise into sticks.
4. Heat oil in a skillet over medium high heat.

5. Sauté tofu until golden brown, then transfer to a large bowl and toss with 2/3 cup of the warm sauce.

6. Sprinkle with sesame seeds and toss lightly. Serve with remaining sauce for dipping.

Quinoa Pilaf

Ingredients

- 1 Tbsp. extra virgin olive oil
- 1 small red onion, chopped
- 1 cup quinoa, rinsed and drained
- 2 cups low sodium vegetable broth
- 1/2 tsp. sea salt
- 2/3 cup dried unsulphured organic cranberries
- 2/3 cup sliced almonds
- 2 Tbsp. hemp seeds

Instructions

1. Heat oil in a medium pot over medium high heat.
2. Add onions and cook, stirring often until just softened-2 to 3 minutes.
3. Add quinoa, stirring constantly for 1 minute.
4. Stir in broth and salt- bring to a boil, then reduce heat to medium low, cover and simmer for 10 minutes.
5. Stir in cranberries, cover again and continue to cook until liquid is completely absorbed and quinoa is tender- 8 to 10 minutes more.
6. Toss with almonds and hemp seeds, then serve.
7. Serving suggestion- serve this over a bed of fresh spinach and arugula, drizzled with extra virgin olive oil and fresh squeezed lemon.

Roasted Veggies with Tempeh, Quinoa and Dried Cranberries

Ingredients

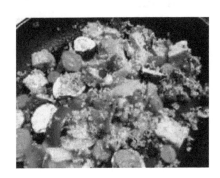

- 1 eggplant, diced
- 1 zucchini, diced
- 1 cup red onion, diced
- 1 cup each red, green and yellow pepper, diced
- 3-4 garlic cloves, whole
- 3 Tbsp. extra virgin olive oil
- 1 tsp. dried oregano
- 1 tsp. dried mint
- 1/4 cup balsamic vinegar
- 1/2 tsp. sea salt
- 1 cup quinoa, cooked
- 3-4 Tbsp. dried organic unsulphured cranberries

Tempeh

- 2 cups tempeh, chopped
- 2 Tbsp. extra virgin olive oil

Instructions

1. Preheat oven to 375°F. In a large bowl, toss all veggies with extra virgin olive oil and dried herbs.

2. Spread on a baking sheet and bake for 20-25 minutes or until veggies are slightly brown and garlic is soft.

3. Place all veggies in a bowl and toss with vinegar and salt.

4. Meanwhile, sauté tempeh in 2 Tbsp. of extra virgin olive oil for 3-4 minutes on each side.

5. Toss veggies with tempeh, quinoa and dried cranberries.

Butternut Squash and Pesto Pizza

Ingredients

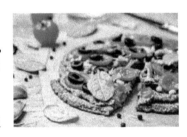

- 1 small butternut squash, peeled, halved and sliced 1/8-inch thick
- 1 medium onion, halved and thinly sliced (1 cup)
- 2 Tbsp. extra virgin olive oil plus more for drizzling
- 2 Tbsp. pesto (recipe below or good quality store bought)
- 1 Tbsp. fresh rosemary, finely chopped
- 2 Gluten free pizza crusts
- 1 cup fresh spinach leaves

Lemon Basil Pesto Ingredients

- 1 cup pine nuts
- 2 - 4 cloves garlic, peeled
- 1 tsp. lemon zest
- ¼ -½ tsp. sea salt
- 3 cups tightly packed fresh basil leaves
- 1/4 cup extra virgin olive oil
- 2 - 4 Tbsp. fresh lemon juice

Pesto Instructions

6. Place the pine nuts, garlic and lemon zest in a food processor fitted with the 'S' blade.

7. Pulse a few times until mixture is coarsely ground. Add fresh basil leaves. While the food processor is running, slowly add in extra virgin olive oil and lemon juice through the tube. Continue to process until the pesto reaches desired consistency.

Pizza Instructions

1. Preheat oven to 400°F.
2. Toss together squash, onion, oil and rosemary in a bowl.
3. Spread onto large baking sheet with parchment paper and roast for 30
4. minutes or until tender.
5. Remove from oven and set aside.
6. Place pizza crusts onto baking sheet. Top with pesto, spinach and squash mixture- add any other toppings you would like.
7. Bake 10-12 minutes or until crust is crisp.

Happy Vegan Bowl

Ingredients

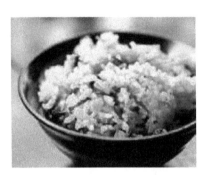

- 2 cups brown rice, cooked
- 1 sweet potato, cooked and cut into chunks
- 1 avocado, diced
- 1 tomato, diced
- 2 Tbsp. red onion, chopped finely
- ¼ cup almonds, roughly chopped
- 2 Tbsp. sunflower seeds
- 2 Tbsp. extra virgin olive oil
- 2 Tbsp. tamari or coconut aminos
- 1 tsp. dried oregano
- 1 tsp. dried basil
- 2 Tbsp. fresh cilantro, chopped
- Black pepper to taste

Instructions

1. Drizzle sweet potato with 1 Tbsp. olive oil and roast at 375°F for 35 minutes. For a quicker option, steam sweet potato in vegetable steamer for 15 minutes.

2. To assemble bowl – add all ingredients into a large bowl and mix together. Feel free to adjust seasonings/dressing to your preference. This dish is so versatile! Add in whichever nuts/seeds you like and get creative by mixing in other vegetables you may have on hand.

The Best Tempeh Vegan Chili

Ingredients

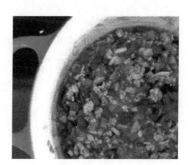

- 1 8oz. package tempeh, crumbled
- 1 large onion, chopped
- 3 large cloves garlic, minced
- 2 Tbsp. extra virgin olive oil or coconut oil for sautéing
- 1 can (15 oz.) red kidney beans, drained and rinsed
- 1 can (28 oz.) fresh diced tomatoes
- 1 can (4 oz.) mild green chilies, diced
- 1 green bell pepper, cored, seeded and diced
- 2 Tbsp. chili powder
- 1/2 tsp. chipotle powder (optional)
- Sea salt and freshly cracked pepper to taste
- 1 cup water
- Scallions, for garnish
- Sliced avocado, for garnish

Instructions

1. In a large Dutch oven or stockpot, heat oil over medium heat.
2. Add onions, garlic, spices and tempeh and cook for 5 minutes, stirring frequently.

3. Add beans, tomatoes, green chilies, bell pepper and water.

4. Bring to a boil, reduce heat to low, partially cover and simmer for roughly 45 minutes.

5. Let sit for 15-20 minutes before serving. Serve with green onions, avocado or cilantro.

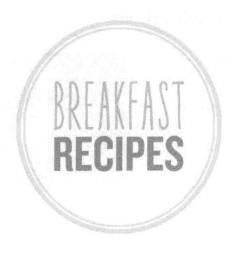

Protein Meal Plan Recipes

Turkey Veggie Frittata

Ingredients

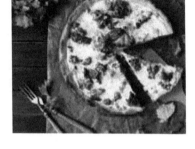

- 8 eggs
- 1lb. ground turkey thigh
- ½ small onion, chopped
- 1 cup mushrooms, sliced
- 2 cups broccoli florets, chopped
- 3-4 sun dried tomatoes, roughly chopped (optional)
- 3 garlic cloves, chopped
- ½ tsp. dried basil
- ½ tsp. dried oregano
- ½ tsp. Cajun spice blend
- ½ smoked paprika
- ½ avocado, sliced
- Sea salt and pepper

Instructions

1. Preheat oven to 350º F. In a bowl, whisk together eggs with basil, Cajun spices, paprika, salt and pepper. Set aside.

2. In a cast iron skillet over medium heat, cook turkey for 5-7 minutes, breaking it up and allowing it to brown.

3. Add in onions, garlic, mushrooms, tomatoes and broccoli and sauté until turkey is browned and no pink remains.

4. Pour in eggs. Allow eggs to cook for 5 minutes, making sure to lift up portions of the egg that have set with a spatula and tilt pan to allow uncooked eggs to run underneath.

5. Once eggs start to set, place skillet in the oven and bake for 15-17 minutes or until no longer runny. You can also turn the broiler on low for the last few minutes to gently brown the top.

6. Serve topped with sliced avocado or serve as a main entrée for dinner with a side salad.

Protein Packed Gluten Free Crepes

Ingredients

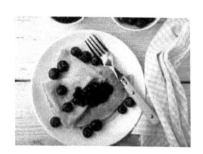

- 4 eggs
- 1 cup unsweetened coconut milk
- 1/2 cup tapioca flour
- 1/2 cup almond flour
- 1/2 tsp. baking powder
- 1/2 tsp. cinnamon
- Pinch of sea salt
- Coconut oil, for oiling pan

Instructions

1. Combine all ingredients into a large bowl (minus the coconut oil) and whisk together until smooth- a few lumps may remain.

2. Heat a small amount of coconut oil in a skillet or crepe pan over medium heat.

3. Add the batter to the pan using a soup ladle or 1/4 cup measuring cup, tilting the pan gently to evenly spread out the batter. You want a thin layer covering your pan. It is like making a large, thin pancake.

4. Cook until the edges start to set, then gently flip and cook on the other side for about 1-2 minutes.

5. Transfer the fresh crepe onto a plate or wire rack to cool and/or eat right away, while still warm. Make remaining

crepes with batter and spread on your favourite toppings such as fresh berries, dried coconut, chopped raw walnuts or pecans.

Chocolate Hazelnut Protein Power Bowl

Ingredients

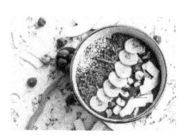

- 1 frozen banana
- ¼ cup hazelnuts, soaked 30 minutes
- 3 Tbsp. hemp seeds
- 2 Tbsp. raw cacao powder
- 1 scoop vanilla vegan protein powder
- ¾ cup unsweetened coconut milk
- 1 tsp. cinnamon
- Ice (optional)
- 1/4 avocado (optional and may be needed for additional thickness and consistency)

Toppings

- Strawberries
- Cacao nibs
- Shredded coconut
- Hemp seeds
- Chia seeds
- Goji berries
- Hazelnuts
- Sesame Seeds
- Pumpkins Seeds

Instructions

1. Place all ingredients (minus the toppings) into a blender and blend until well combined.

2. Pour into a bowl and top with your favorite ingredients. Topping with hemp seeds, chia seeds and other superfoods will give this bowl a super antioxidant kick and supply you with a ton of plant based protein and healthy fats.

Energizing Blueberry Spinach Smoothie

Ingredients

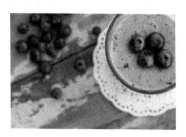

- 1/2 cup frozen blueberries
- 1/4 avocado for creaminess
- 2 large handfuls of organic spinach
- 2 cups coconut water
- 1 cup unsweetened almond, coconut or cashew milk
- 1 scoop vanilla vegan protein powder
- 1 Tbsp. chia seeds
- 3-4 ice cubes (optional)
- 1 tsp. cinnamon

Instructions

1. Blend together in a high speed blender.

Veggie Egg Muffins

Ingredients

- 1/2 tsp. coconut oil
- 1/2 medium onion, chopped
- 1/4 red pepper, chopped
- 8 eggs
- Sea salt and pepper to taste

Instructions

1. Preheat oven to 400°F.
2. Grease muffin tin with coconut oil.
3. Rinse and chop all veggies into 1/4 inch pieces. Divide vegetables evenly between muffin tins.
4. Whisk the eggs, then pour into tins, dividing it evenly.
5. Sprinkle with salt and pepper, then stir the vegetable and egg mixture briefly to evenly disperse the vegetables throughout the egg.
6. Bake for 18-20 minutes.

Coco-No-Oat Granola

Ingredients

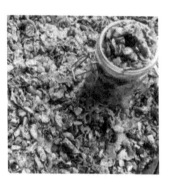

- 3 cups coconut flakes, unsweetened
- 1 cup pecans, roughly chopped
- ½ cup pumpkin seeds
- ½ cup almonds, roughly chopped
- 2 Tbsp. chia seeds
- 2 tsp. cinnamon
- 5-6 Tbsp. coconut oil, melted
- 2 tsp. maple syrup

Instructions

1. Preheat oven to 250°F and line a baking sheet with parchment paper.
2. Combine all ingredients in a large bowl, then spread evenly on a tray. (You could use 2 trays or 1 large one).
3. Bake for 20-30 minutes, until golden and desired crispness is reached. Be sure to remove it from the oven halfway and stir gently.

Vanilla Maple Chia Pudding

Ingredients

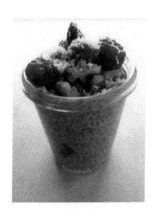

- 3/4 cup chia seeds
- 4 cups unsweetened almond or coconut milk
- 1/2 tsp. ground vanilla bean
- 1 tsp. cinnamon
- 2 tsp. maple syrup
- Pinch of sea salt

Instructions

1. In a large mason jar, add all your ingredients.
2. Secure jar with lid and give it a good shake. Alternatively, you can add everything to a blender and blend together for a few seconds, then pour into the mason jar.
3. Leave in fridge overnight.
4. In the morning, shake again really well, then pour out desired serving into a bowl.
5. Top with your favourite superfood ingredients!

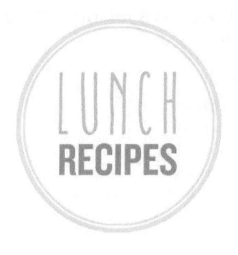

Protein Meal Plan Recipes

Green Goodness Bowl with Dill Hummus Dressing

Ingredients

- ½ cup hummus
- ½ lemon, juiced
- 1 Tbsp. extra virgin olive oil
- ½ cup fresh dill
- Sea salt and black pepper (to taste)
- 1 Tbsp. coconut oil
- 8 cups kale leaves
- 1 zucchini, diced
- 1 cup frozen edamame, thawed
- 1 cup frozen peas, thawed
- ½ cup raw cashews
- 1 avocado, sliced
- 2 chicken breasts, diced
- 4 green onions, chopped

Instructions

1. In a jar, combine hummus, lemon juice, olive oil and dill. Season with sea salt and black pepper. Shake well and set aside. You may need to add 1 Tbsp. of warm water to thin it depending on the consistency of your hummus.

2. Heat coconut oil in a large pan over medium heat. Add kale, zucchini and sauté until kale is just wilted. Remove from heat and set aside.

3. Divide kale and zucchini between bowls and top with edamame, green peas, green onions, chicken and avocado. Drizzle with dill hummus dressing.

Rainbow Collard Wraps

Ingredients

- ¼ cup Hummus
- 4 large collard green leaves
- 2 cups chicken breast thinly sliced or ground turkey
- ½ cup red pepper, thinly sliced
- ½ cup shredded red cabbage
- ½ cup grated beets
- ½ cup grated carrots
- ¼ cup green onions, finely chopped

Instructions

1. Lay collard greens flat on a cutting board and remove the stems, keeping the leaves connected at the top.
2. Spread 1-2 Tbsp. of hummus on each leaf.
3. Top with chicken or turkey. Layer the vegetables on top.
4. Wrap each collard leaf like a burrito, folding the bottom up first and then the sides. Continue to roll until all the contents are tucked inside.

Tuna Toss Up

Ingredients

- 1 can water pack tuna mixed
- ½ cup grated carrot
- ½ cup grated apple
- ½ squeezed lemon
- 2 Tbsp. apple cider vinegar
- 1 Tbsp. dill weed
- 1 Tbsp. extra virgin olive oil
- Sea salt and black pepper

Instructions

1. Combine all ingredients into a bowl and enjoy!

Detox Green Salad with Pumpkin Seeds and Chicken

Ingredients

- 4 cups mixed salad greens
- 2 stalks celery, diced finely
- 1 cucumber, peeled and diced
- 1 cup sunflower sprouts, cut into 1 inch pieces
- 1 avocado, diced
- 1 cup raw pumpkin seeds
- 2 Tbsp. apple cider vinegar or lemon juice
- 1/3 cup extra virgin olive oil
- Himalayan sea salt, to taste
- Black pepper to taste
- 1 tsp. dried thyme
- 1 tsp. Dijon mustard

Instructions

1. Combine the salad greens, cucumber, celery, avocado and sprouts together in a salad bowl. Sprinkle the pumpkin seeds on top.
2. Mix the olive oil, apple cider vinegar, mustard, salt, pepper and thyme together in a small bowl.
3. Drizzle over salad.
4. Top with leftover Roasted Lemon Rosemary Chicken.

Kale Salad

Ingredients
Salad

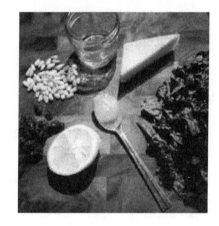

- 1 large bunch kale, washed, de-stemmed and broken up into pieces
- 1/4 cup pine nuts
- 1/3 cup organic sulphite free dried cranberries
- 1 Tbsp. nutritional yeast (optional)

Dressing

- 3-4 Tbsp. extra virgin olive oil
- 1 Tbsp. raw honey
- Juice of 1 lemon

Instructions

1. Mix dressing ingredients in a bowl using a whisk. The honey is quite sticky, so it may require a few minutes of stirring and whisking.
2. Add all salad ingredients to a large bowl and add in dressing. Allow salad to sit for 5-10 minutes to allow the kale to slightly wilt and absorb the dressing.
3. Serve with leftover meatloaf muffins.

Green Egg White Scramble

Ingredients

- 1 cup egg whites or 3 egg whites plus 1 whole egg
- ½ cup asparagus, diced
- ½ cup red peppers, diced
- 2 cups spinach, chopped
- ½ cup cherry tomatoes, halved
- 1 tsp. coconut oil
- Sea salt and black pepper, to taste

Instructions

1. Combine all ingredients and mix well.
2. Add coconut oil to sauté pan. Add egg mixture and cook 5-7 minutes on medium heat.
3. Serve and enjoy.

Apple Quinoa Salad

Ingredients

- 1 cup cooked quinoa
- 1/2 cup chopped walnuts
- 1/2 small red bell pepper, chopped
- 1/3 cup red onion, chopped
- 1/2 cup fresh parsley, chopped
- 1/4 cup lemon juice
- 2 - 3 Tbsp. vegetable broth (see recipe)
- Salt and pepper to taste
- 1/4 tsp. cinnamon
- 1 clove minced garlic
- 1 large chopped apple

Instructions

1. Make sure the quinoa is cooled before starting this recipe.
2. Mix all ingredients except for the quinoa, walnuts and apple.
3. Once combined, add the quinoa, walnuts and apple, then mix well.

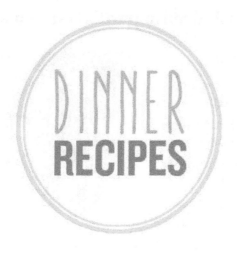

Protein Meal Plan
Recipes

Garlic Chili Shrimp with Pesto Zoodles

Ingredients

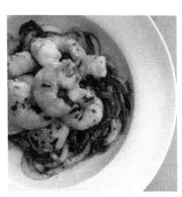

- 2 large zucchinis, spiralized
- 1 large bag frozen shrimp, defrosted
- 2 cloves fresh garlic, minced
- 1 tsp. chili flakes (or more if you like it hot)
- 2 Tbsp. fresh parsley, roughly chopped
- Black pepper
- Extra virgin olive oil, for sautéing

Instructions

1. Spiralize zucchini and set aside.
2. Defrost shrimp and remove shells.
3. Add extra virgin olive oil to large sauté pan. Once hot, add in shrimp, garlic, chili flakes, parsley and black pepper.
4. Cook for 2-3 minutes on each side until cooked through and nicely pink. Remove from the skillet and place in a bowl.
5. In the same skillet, add in zucchini noodles and cook for roughly 4-5 minutes until desired texture is reached.
6. Add noodles to a bowl and top with shrimp and fresh parsley.
7. Enjoy!

Cauliflower Fried Rice

Ingredients

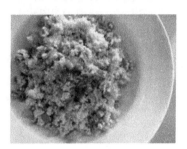

- 1 large cauliflower head
- 2 large eggs, beaten
- 1 Tbsp. minced ginger
- 3 garlic cloves, minced
- 2 medium carrots, diced
- ½ cup peas, fresh or frozen
- ½ onion, chopped
- 4 green onions, thinly sliced
- ¼ cup cashews, optional
- 3 Tbsp. coconut amino or gluten free tamari
- 1 tsp. chili flakes
- Sea salt and pepper
- Coconut oil, for sautéing

Instructions

1. Cut the cauliflower into florets, discarding the tough inner core. Working in batches, pulse the cauliflower in a food processor until it breaks down into rice-sized pieces.

2. Heat a large skillet over medium heat and drizzle in coconut oil. Add onion, carrots and sauté until tender-about 2 minutes. Add in ginger, garlic and stir together.

3. Slide veggie mixture to one side of the skillet and add in the beaten eggs, scrambling until cooked through and then mix with the veggies.

4. Stir in cauliflower "rice" and peas and mix everything together well. Add in coconut aminos. Cook for 6 to 8 minutes, until cauliflower is soft and tender. Add in chili flakes, sea salt and pepper.

5. Top with green onions and cashews- serve and enjoy!

Roasted Lemon Rosemary Chicken with Wild Green Salad

Ingredients-Chicken

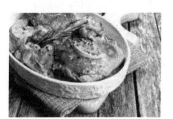

- 4 organic boneless, skinless chicken breasts
- 2 Tbsp. Dijon mustard
- 1 tsp. grainy mustard
- 2 sprigs fresh rosemary, chopped
- 2 sprigs fresh thyme
- 2 Tbsp. extra virgin olive oil
- Juice of half a lemon
- Sea salt and fresh pepper

Instructions-Chicken

1. Preheat oven to 350° F. Place chicken in a large bowl and add in all ingredients (sprigs should be removed from fresh herbs).

2. Using your hands, mix together really well. Place bowl in the fridge and let sit for 20 minutes to marinade.

3. Cook chicken for 35 minutes on baking sheet covered with parchment paper. Turn oven to low broil and cook another 10 minutes until skin is nice and crispy and fully cooked through.

4. Serve this alongside a large salad for a simple detox meal.

Ingredients- Wild Green Salad

- 2 cups wild greens
- ½ med apple diced
- ¼ cup diced celery
- ½ cup grated carrot
- ½ lemon

Instructions

1. Toss all ingredients into a bowl except lemon.
2. Squeeze lemon over salad and enjoy.

Meatloaf Muffins

Ingredients
Muffins

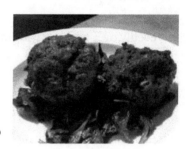

- 2 organic eggs
- 1 can organic tomato paste
- 1/2 Tbsp. dried oregano
- 1 tsp. dried rosemary
- 1 tsp. dried thyme
- 1 tsp. sea salt
- 1/2 tsp. of hot sauce
- 2 lbs. organic ground beef or ground turkey
- 1 cup gluten free rolled oats
- 1 large onion, finely chopped

Topping

- 1/4 cup tomato sauce
- 1 Tbsp. organic Dijon mustard
- 1 Tbsp. prepared horseradish (optional)

Instructions

1. Preheat oven to 375°F.
2. Lightly grease a muffin pan.
3. Lightly whisk eggs in large bowl. Whisk in tomato paste, herbs and hot sauce.
4. Add ground beef or turkey, oats and onions. Using your hands, thoroughly blend everything together. Evenly

place the seasoned ground beef or turkey into the muffin cups.

5. Whisk together the topping ingredients and brush evenly over the meaty muffin tops.

6. Bake for 25-30 minutes, or until cooked through. Serve and Enjoy!

Spaghetti Squash Bake with Italian Sausage and Herbs

Ingredients

- 1 large spaghetti squash
- 1 lb. hormone and antibiotic free turkey sausage
- 1 small yellow onion, diced
- 1 cup tomato sauce- no sugar added
- 1 tsp. dried basil
- 1 tsp. dried oregano
- ½ tsp. chili flakes
- Sea salt and pepper, to taste
- 3 eggs, whisked
- 1 red pepper, chopped

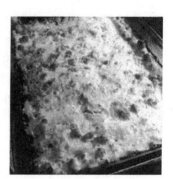

Instructions

1. Preheat oven to 400°F degrees.
2. Cut spaghetti squash in half lengthwise. Place spaghetti squash cut side down on a baking sheet lined with parchment paper and bake for 20-25 minutes or until the skin of the squash becomes slightly soft and you can puncture it with a fork. Remove squash from oven and reduce oven heat to 350°F.
3. Remove squash using a fork, scrape down the squash to form spaghetti and place in an 8×8 greased baking dish.

4. Place a large pan over medium heat. Add sausage, red pepper and onion. Break sausage up into pieces and cook until pink no longer remains.

5. Add pizza sauce, dried herbs, spices and salt and pepper to the pan and mix well.

6. Add sausage mixture to the 8×8 baking dish and mix well with spaghetti squash.

7. Lastly, add whisked eggs to the baking dish and mix everything together well until you can no longer see the eggs.

8. Place in oven and bake for 1 hour or until the top of the mixture forms a slight crust. It will look as though the top layer is covered with cheese!

9. Let rest for 5 minutes before serving.

10. Optional- top with chopped fresh basil. Enjoy!

Coconut Ginger Salmon with Roasted Asparagus

Ingredients

- 1/2 onion, diced
- 1 Tbsp. coconut oil
- 1 Tbsp. ginger root, grated
- ½ tsp. ground fennel
- ½ tsp. cinnamon
- 1 cup coconut milk
- 1 Tbsp. lemon juice
- ½ Tbsp. lemon zest
- 1/3 lb. wild salmon
- ¼ cup fresh cilantro, chopped or 1-2 tsp. dried
- Himalayan sea salt, to taste

Instructions

1. Sauté the onion in the oil until onions are translucent, about 8 minutes. Add the ginger, spices and cook for another 2 minutes.
2. Add the coconut milk, lemon juice and zest and stir to combine. Place the whole fish fillet into the sauce and cook over low heat for about 7-10 minutes or until fish flakes away with a fork at the thickest part.
3. Garnish with chopped cilantro and salt to taste.

Roasted Asparagus with Walnuts

Ingredients

- 1 bunch asparagus
- 1 Tbsp. extra virgin olive oil
- 1 Tbsp. balsamic vinegar
- 1 Tbsp. fresh squeezed lemon juice
- Pinch sea salt
- Black pepper
- ½ cup walnuts

Instructions

1. Preheat oven to 375°F.
2. Spread asparagus onto a pan lined with parchment paper.
3. Mix extra virgin olive oil, balsamic, lemon juice, salt and pepper together.
4. Pour mixture over asparagus, mix well.
5. Roast in oven for approximately 15 minutes.
6. Top with walnuts and serve.

Slow Cooker Whole Roasted Chicken

Ingredients

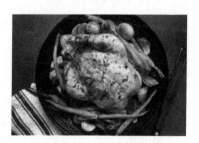

- 4-6 lb whole chicken
- 2 ½ cups chicken or vegetable broth
- 1 lemon, cut in half
- 1 large bunch fresh thyme
- 1 large carrot, roughly chopped
- 1 celery stalk, roughly chopped
- 1 onion, chopped into 4 parts
- 3 garlic cloves, crushed, left whole with skin on
- 2 Tbsp. extra virgin olive oil
- 2-3 Tbsp. dried Italian herbs or mixture of your favourite dried herbs. Oregano, thyme, rosemary, parsley, savoury etc.
- Sea salt and pepper

Instructions

1. Prepare chicken. Remove giblets and neck or ask your butcher to do this for you.
2. Place the lemon, fresh thyme and ¼ of the onion inside the cavity of the chicken.
3. Add sea salt, pepper, dried herbs and extra virgin olive oil onto chicken. Rub this all over the chicken. Spread this generously all over. If you feel you need to add more herbs or extra virgin olive oil, do so. This depends on

the size of your chicken. The ingredient amounts above work well for 4-6 lbs.

4. Place into your crockpot, add chopped carrots, celery, garlic and leftover onion.

5. Place the chicken breast side up into the crock pot and add in chicken stock.

6. Turn your crockpot onto the low setting for 8 hours.

7. After 8 hours, let your chicken sit for at least 15-20 minutes before carving.

8. Serve with a side of roasted veggies or salad.

9. If you prefer to have a crisper chicken, remove the chicken from the crock pot after it's cooked and place it into a roasting pan. Put it in the oven at 425°F and cook for 5-10 minutes or until reaching desired crispness.

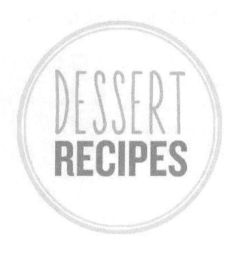

Bonus Dessert Recipes

During the 10-Day Detox, the following dessert recipes are acceptable as well as delicious! Treat yourself! Enjoy!

Almond Vanilla Protein Clusters

Ingredients

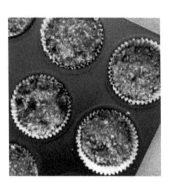

- 1 cup raw almonds
- 1 cup raw pumpkin seeds
- 2 tsp. ground cinnamon
- 1 tsp. ground ginger
- 1/2 tsp. sea salt
- 1 cup unsweetened shredded coconut
- 1/2 cup Thompson raisins
- 1/2 cup raw almond butter
- 2 scoops vanilla protein powder
- 2 Tbsp. maple syrup
- 1/4 cup unsweetened applesauce

Instructions

1. Line a muffin pan with paper liners and set aside.
2. In a food processor fitted with the S blade, process the almonds, pumpkin seeds, cinnamon, ginger and sea salt until finely chopped. Transfer the mixture to a large bowl.
3. Stir in the coconut and raisins.
4. In a small saucepan over medium heat, melt together the almond butter, protein powder, maple syrup and applesauce. When mixture is smooth and combined, pour over nut mix.

5. Stir together until all nuts are evenly coated and thoroughly mixed.

6. Divide the mixture evenly in the 12 muffin cups. You may need to slightly wet your hands in order to press the mixture down into the cups and keep your fingers from sticking.

7. Eat as is or store in the fridge to cool. Clusters can be stored in an airtight container in the fridge or freezer.

No Bake Apple Bites

Ingredients

- 1 cup oats (quick or traditional)
- 4 Tbsp. ground flax seed
- 1/2 tsp. cinnamon
- 1/3 cup almond butter
- 1 Tbsp. maple syrup
- 1 apple (peeled, cored and finely diced)

Instructions

1. Combine oats, ground flaxseed and cinnamon together in a bowl. Mix well. Add almond butter, maple syrup and diced apples. Mix well again.
2. Roll the dough into balls, about the size of a golf ball.
3. Wet hands before rolling to prevent sticking.
4. Place the bites on a plate and let sit in the fridge for at least 30 minutes to firm.
5. Then transfer into an airtight container and store in the fridge for 3 to 4 days. Enjoy!

Raw Cacao Energy Bites

Ingredients

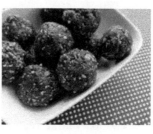

- 1 cup walnuts
- 1/4 cup sunflower seeds
- 2 Tbsp. hemp seeds
- 1/4 cup raw cacao powder
- 12 pitted medjool dates
  (soaked in water for 5 minutes to soften)
- 1 tsp. vanilla powder
- 1/4 tsp. sea salt

Instructions

1. Add all ingredients, except dates, into a food processor and pulse to break up the nuts and seeds. Then add in dates and blend until mixture sticks together.
2. Using your hands, roll into balls and place onto a parchment lined dish.
3. Place in the fridge for 15 minutes to slightly harden.
4. These will last about 1 week in the fridge.

Chocolate Matcha Balls

Ingredients

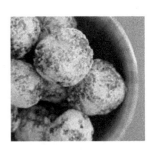

- 7 medjool dates, pitted
- ½ cup whole raw almonds
- ¼ cup unsweetened cocoa powder
- 1 scoop vanilla vegan protein powder
- 1 Tbsp. cacao nibs
- 1 Tbsp. matcha powder, plus more for rolling*
- 1 tsp. ground vanilla
- 1 tsp. ground cinnamon
- 2 Tbsp. maple syrup

Instructions

1. Place all ingredients into a food processor and pulse until well combined.
2. Roll 'dough' into roughly 1-inch balls about the size of a Tbsp. and place onto a plate.
3. In a bowl, add about 3-4 tsp. of matcha powder.
4. Roll balls into powder and place back onto plate, then eat and enjoy!
5. Store in the refrigerator for 7 days.

Nut and Seed Raw Granola Bars

Ingredients

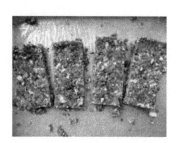

- 3 large medjool dates
- 1 cup raw almonds
- 1 cup raw walnuts
- 1/4 cup hemp seeds
- 1/4 cup sunflower seeds
- 1/4 cup pumpkin seeds
- 1/4 cup chia seeds
- 1/2 cup almond butter
- 1/4 cup maple syrup
- 1 tsp. ground vanilla bean
- 1 tsp. ground cinnamon

Instructions

1. Combine all ingredients into a food processor and process until smooth.
2. Scoop mixture into an 8x8 brownie pan prepared with parchment paper and press down to flatten.
3. Refrigerate for 30 minutes to firm up.
4. Cut in 12 or 16 bars.

CPSIA information can be obtained
at www.ICGtesting.com
Printed in the USA
LVHW05s1323110418
573008LV00001B/1/P

9 781545 625262